Copyright © 2010 by Watson Enterprises LLC All rights reserved No part of this publication may be reproduced, stored in a retrieval system, or transmitted in any form or by any means, electronic, mechanical, photocopying, recording, scanning, or otherwise, except as permitted under Section 107 or 108 of the 1976 United States Copyright Act, without either the prior written permission of the Publisher, or authorization through payment of the appropriate per-copy fee to the Copyright Clearance Center.

Limit of Liability/Disclaimer of Warranty: This book is designed to provide information about the subject matter.

It is sold with the understanding that the publisher and authors are not engaged in rendering legal, coaching or other professional services.

While the publisher and author have used their best efforts in preparing this book, they make no representations or warranties with respect to the accuracy or completeness of the contents of this book and specifically disclaim any implied warranties of merchantability or fitness for a particular purpose.
No warranty may be created or extended by sales representatives or written sales materials. This book is not intended or should be a substitute for therapy or professional advice.

The views and opinions expressed in this page are strictly those of the author. The advice and strategies contained herein may not be suitable for your situation.

The publisher is not engaged in rendering professional services, and you should consult a competent professional where appropriate.

Neither the publisher nor author shall be liable for any loss of profit or any other commercial damages, including but not limited to special, incidental, consequential, or other damages. This document is provided for educational purposes only.

The reader assumes all risk and responsibility for the usage of any information or ideas contained in this guide. If you do not wish to be bound by the above, you may return the book to the publisher for a full refund

Table of Contents

Introduction	8
Colin's Story of Total Transformation	13
Jayne's Personal Story	21
Why & How HCG Body for Life Weight Loss System Works	32
What Is The HCG Diet?	33
Burn The Fat and Reveal The Muscles	33
How HCG Prevents Hunger Pains	34
HCG Targets the Root Cause of Weight Gain	34
HCG Increases Your Energy By Burning Fat	35
HCG Had No Common Diet Side Effects	35
HCG Weight Loss Clinical Study	36
The Need for Increased Protein Portions	40
The Mental Aspect of The Diet	50
Motivation	51
Previous Failed Diet Attempts	54
Stress	56
The HCG Protocol Explained	64
HCG Diet Original vs. New Advanced HCG Weight Loss System Explained	69
Advanced HCG Weight Loss System	

Comparison Chart	70
Medication	72
Injection Procedure	75
How Much HCG to Inject and How to Fill the Syringe	78

Phases Of The HCG Diet — **81**

Mastering HCG BFL Diet - Gorge-Phase 1	82
Mastering HCG BFL Diet - Fat Loss-Phase 2	84
Mastering HCG BFL Diet - Maintaince-Phase 3	101
Mastering HCG BFL Diet - Life-Phase 4	116

Food & Supplement Choices — **137**

Introduction	137
Foods You Can Eat	138
Foods To Avoid	140
How Much Food Is Allowed?	142
Supplements	145
Recommended Supplements	145
Laminine	146
Acetyl-L-Carnitine	147
Ancient Tea	152
Vitamins and Minerals	158
Vitamin C	160
Vitamin E	160

Sample HCG Diet Menu — **163**

Oriental Ginger Chicken	163
Chicken Tarragon	164
Chicken Cacciatore	165
Meatloaf	166
Ground Beef Tacos	167
Final Words & FAQ	**169**
How To Breakthrough Your HCG Diet Weight Loss Plateau VLOG	170
Why Do Men Lose Weight Faster?	170
HCG Diet Hunger Pains...Is This Normal?	172
HCD Body for Life HIIT Workout System	**173-179**
Acknowledgement	**180**

HCG Body for Life

HCG Body for Life fat loss system is for anyone looking for rapid sustainable weight loss. An easy to follow diet plan to lose fat, build muscle, reshape your body and reveal your true body within.

To your success,

Colin and Jayne

Introduction

The only limitations for your life are the limiting beliefs in your mind

　　　　　　　　　　　　　　　- Matt Morris

You're searching the web and you come across another weight loss diet that promises miraculous weight loss in which you supposedly don't have to exercise, and you'll lose 1 to 2 pounds a day. But the catch is that you have to maintain a 500-calorie diet, eat only certain foods, and if you cheat, you'll actually gain weight. It further promises that you will never regain the weight you lose.

What goes through your mind? You say to yourself "Yeah right"....... Am I right?
Well you are not alone. I did the very same thing, thought the very same thoughts, and the only thing that may be different between you and me is...

At the time I was introduced to this information, I was OPEN, I was WIDE OPEN, I had just spent about an hour sobbing in my closet, and I had surrendered! At that very moment, I stopped looking at myself with disgust and anger, and accepted responsibility for where I was in my life, what I had done to myself, and set out to make a change.

I was done being fat! I was done looking and feeling the way I felt! I was determined to find a solution.

I know you are skeptical right now, and that's ok. I know exactly how you feel. I know that so many diets have failed you in the past. Or maybe you failed them, which was also true for me. Why is this time different? This time is different because I have done all of the legwork for you. I have done all of the experimentation, I have tested what works and what doesn't and I'm going to show you exactly what to do to get the weight off and keep it off. I have laid it out for you step by step.

You see I'm a real person, who has already walked the walk, and I am living proof that this protocol works miracles. Look at my picture, there's no "photo alteration" going on here. I got real results with the process and principles Jayne and I are sharing with you in this book.

And the crazy thing is, with the HCG body for life protocol, I already know what your end result will be before you do. I have had the honor of personally seeing and hearing success story after success story of hundreds of people who got the same results we did from this protocol.

I want you to suspend all doubt and create within you a knowing that this is it! This is the moment that your life is going to change from the inside out.

Now bare with me one more second, I want you to read the next paragraph first, then close your eyes; go ahead close them. I want you to picture a time when you looked the best you ever looked, and felt the best you ever felt and hold that picture in your mind's eye... Remember it, and embrace these feelings; because this is the picture of and image of yourself that you will be able to recreate within the next 26 to 43 days with this weight loss protocol.

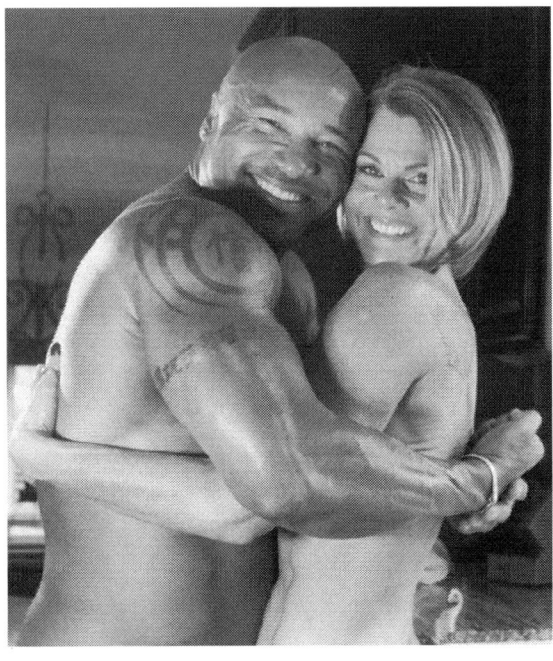

How I look today, mirrors physically the way I looked in my twenties, taking away the aging process. I am in equal shape, I feel as good, and almost as strong, as I did then, and no longer worry about my weight or health.

Common and join Jayne and me on this journey. Take back your life, your health and vitality, it does not matter if you're 15 or 50, man or woman, old or young you can go back while living your future and reveal your true body within.

In the next 26 to 43 days you will discover that feeling good in your own skin, looking in the mirror, and liking what you see is absolutely possible. You're about to know firsthand HCG Body for Life in 26 days. Congratulations on your decision to take back control of your life, your health, and your body!

We are very proud of you, and you should be proud of yourself!

To Your Success, and God Bless,
Colin and Jayne

Therapeutic Uses of HCG

Men

• HCG is used for the treatment of hypogonadism (quite low testosterone) by stimulating the testes to develop far more testosterone by natural means. It naturally raises testosterone levels in men.

Woman

• HCG therapy is employed to treat infertility in high doses by stimulating ovulation and permits for the last maturation of eggs.

• Throughout early pregnancy if the mother does not eat comfortable to nourish the fetus, the HCG will assist offer satisfactory nourishment by obtaining energy from the mother's fat reserves and feed the infant via the placenta.

Mechanism of HCG for Weight loss

Men

• Raised testosterone levels may cause an increase in metabolic process and muscle mass.

• The HCG hormone stimulates the hypothalamus in the to release abnormal fat reserves once on low calorie diet plan is implemented.

• Spares lean muscle tissue

• The body will produce far more energy to burn fat

immediately after the HCG Body for life protocol has been completed.

• Men achieve far more fat loss than women due to their larger quantity of muscle mass.

Woman

• Raised hormone levels on modest scale resulting in an elevated metabolic process.

• The HCG hormone stimulates the hypothalamus in the brain to release abnormal fat reserves once on low calorie diet plan is implemented

• Spares lean muscle tissue

Average Weight loss Results for Females in 6 weeks

• Woman who carefully follow the HCG Body for Life Diet may get rid of on 25-35lbs in 40 days. Equal to ½- ¾ of a pound a day.

Supporting Factors:

* Females of childbearing age have a tendency to get rid of far more weight owing to higher metabolic and hormone levels than menopausal women. Regular reduction may array from <robust>30-35robust> lbs.

* Medical hysterectomy and menopausal patients may get rid of as much as 25r lbs.

Average Weight loss Results for Men in 6 weeks

• Men who carefully follow the HCG Body for Life Diet Protocol may get rid of 35 to 50 lbs. in 4o days.

• About 1 to 1.25 pound a day

Supporting Factors:

• Men in normal possess a higher metabolic rate than women and far more slim muscle.

• A modest increase in testosterone growth may assist elevate the metabolic rate

• Metabolic Behavior

HCG is considered to bring about re-calibration of the hypothalamus gland stabilizes the thyroid, metabolic rate, adrenal glands and storage of fat, to release and mobilize saved vitamins and nutrients inside of the fat cells by shrinking and draining the fat cell's contents.

• The liquefied vitamins and nutrients extracted from the fat stores, are launched into the bloodstream for the body to make use of as energy.

• It is considered that more than 2,000 calories of fat energy may be released into the body in a solitary day, as a result reducing starvation, increasing energy and metabolic process.

My Transformation Story

Before you dive into main content of this book, I'd like to quickly share my own transformation story with you, so you know that it is possible and that I also know first hand how you feel right now, and how you're going to feel once you successfully complete our program. I believe that once you have read my story, you will see that if I can do it, anyone can – including you.

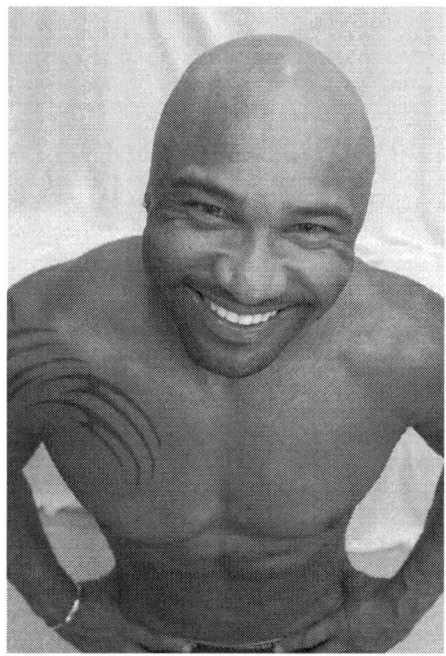

I completed the HCG Diet Protocol almost two years ago. I saw an infomercial for Kevin Trudeau's weight loss cure book at a stage in my life where I'd put on a great deal of weight. My wife

Jayne was very diligent with me and helped me with different weight loss programs.

I was a high school athlete I had always been in great shape and was even voted best body in my high school greatest grads competition. I had never experienced any kind of obesity issues as a young man, nor while in my late twenties early thirties.

Like many of you the years went by and I put on over 40 pounds of fat and went from having a 31inch waist to a 42-inch waist. I already had high blood pressure, but with the excess weight, I also had sleep apnea, and was a borderline diabetic. I could not run half of a mile without being in physical pain and gasping for air.

I tried everything I could but I could not get the weight off no matter what I did. I tried counting calories, nationally known diets that had pre-package food portions; I've counted points, and calories. I did colon cleanses, low carb diets, diet foods, diet detox, lemonade diet. I tried running, working out five to six days a week, any program you can name that claimed to help you lose weight fast. You name it… I tried it.

I was in my closet one day putting on a suit to go to work; and I couldn't get any of my pants to button. For some reason at that moment it just hit me like a ton of bricks that I had gained so much weight that I could no longer wear my own cloths, and I began to cry. I realized that my life and my weight were out of control and I just broke down into tears.

It was at that time that I became committed to doing whatever it was going to take to overcome my weight issues.

If you enjoy the process, it's your dream. If you are enduring it, desperate for the result, it's somebody else's ~ LOA

When I came across this so-called weight loss cure. I was very skeptical about it. My wife Jayne had a little more confidence in the diet protocol due to a past experience with a similar diet when she was in her 20's, so we decided to give it a try.

To cut a long story short, I lost 41 pounds in 43 days and completely reshaped my body. As such, that opened up a new journey and a quest for me to acquire as much knowledge about health and fitness as possible so I could help others pursue lifelong health. Success came in many forms for me. The protocol, corrected my blood pressure, stabilized my blood sugar, corrected the sleep apnea disorder and allowed me to stop taking my high blood pressure medication that had been taking for more than 20 years.

My health problems and pre-diabetic condition simply vanished. I come from a family history whereby both of my parents and paternal grandparents are all diseased from heart disease or diabetes related organ failure. As you can see, it was more than just my body image on the line for me.

This protocol definitely changed my life, corrected my health problems, and opened up new opportunities for me to share my journey and passions to rid the world of obesity; especially among the African American communities where diabetes, high blood pressure, and obesity are at epidemic proportions. I am now on a mission to help other people all over the world achieve and even surpass my results with this amazing fat loss breakthrough.

Jayne and I made some core tweaks to the original Dr. Simons protocol that we feel strongly about. You will discover within these pages, the subtle but powerful changes that were made that helped up both pack on pounds of lean muscle, and lose tons of body fat. When I began my journey I had a body mass index (BMI) of 34 percent. We I concluded the HCG Body for Life protocol implementing our core tweaks to the protocol I had a BMI of 8.9 percent.

With that said, I just want you to know that I'm a real person who has experienced real results like thousands, if not millions of people from across the globe. I am honored to be presenting this information to you, and am glad that you're taking the time to take your life back by reading this book.

I know that by giving you this information it's going to change your life, and make completing this protocol much easier for you, and guarantee your success.

"You have to believe it before you see it" Dr. Wayne Dyer

This is my promise to you... **YOU WILL BECOME A BELIEVER** within the first **96 hours** of the HCG Body for Life Protocol. Give yourself 96 hours, and you will **NEVER** worry about being overweight or obese again. I guarantee it!

I coined three types of reasons that people have for using this diet. Some people can experience all three phases like I did, but usually there are 3 main reasons.

1. To get some weight off and find something that works to lose the weight.

2. To really improve your looks, and have a goal in mind to fit into a certain size or look a certain way based on how you looked in the past.

3. You truly want to completely transform your body.

The HCG Body for Life system will definitely get you to each and every stage of the above options, you will just need to decide how far you want take it.

I've got to tell you that I went through all three stages as I began to believe it was possible. In the beginning, the first stage for me was just, "I've got to get some weight off so I can just fit into my clothes."

As I saw the weight coming off, I realized that there was a real possibility that I would actually start seeing my abs for the first time in 15 years. I thought, "Well wait; now I want to be able to get down to a 32 or 34-inch pair of jeans, which to me was a really huge quest.

When that became possible and all of a sudden I realized I had six-pack abs and I started looking really fit, the next level was… I wanted to completely transform my body and look like a fitness model, if that's even possible at 48 years old. Guess what, I think I am really close. And the thing that is so amazing about this protocol is your vision changes as you realize what is now possible for you.

This diet is actually not new. It's been around since 1954. A doctor named A.T.W. Simeons discovered that if you use a small amount of this hormone called HCG (which stands for human chorionic gonadotropin) with a very low calorie diet it would actually create massive and fast weight loss.

He also discovered that HCG targeted your abnormal fat stores. We have normal fat that protects our muscles and organs and we also have the abnormal fat that goes into all those other places in our body. You know those areas of the body we all hate. And that no matter how much we diet, exercise and starve ourselves to lose weight, some of those areas never go away.

You always have one area that starts to look good, but the rest of your body doesn't seem to get fixed. Dr. Simeons discovered that HCG would basically attack and release all of the abnormal fat in the body and use that released fat as energy. By using the released fat you are able to sustain low calorie diet for long periods of time.

Some people believe that if you just did a 500-calorie diet without HCG you would lose the weight anyway. Now, part of that is true.

Yes, you would lose some weight in the very beginning, but very quickly within a week to 10 days, you'd start to feel very weak, irritable, and lifeless, suffer from headaches, and have no energy because your body would go into starvation mode due to the lack of enough food to sustain you.

HCG releases 3,000 to 5,000 and sometimes 7,000 calories of fat into your blood stream for you to use as energy. You actually have more than enough energy to go about your normal life and you're not hungry. And that was the miracle of this diet. You can actually eat a sensible diet, a 500-calorie (low calorie diet) and not be hungry throughout the day.

Jayne's Personal Story

"Hold up your hands before your eyes. You are looking at the hands of God."
By Rabbi Lawrence Kushner

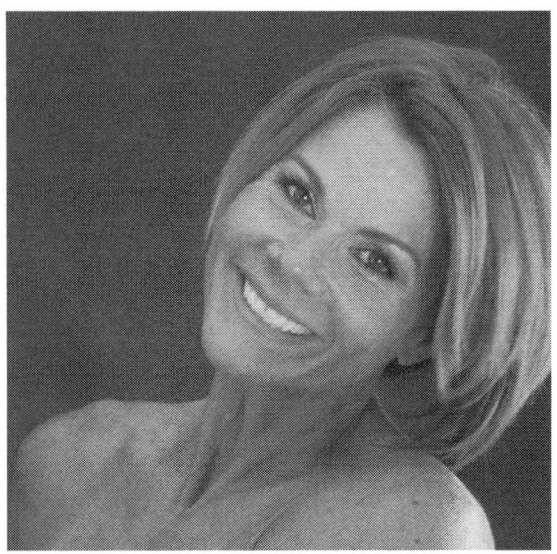

Thank you Colin for this amazing journey I have had and am on with you...I would not be who I am or where I am today without you in my life...I love you with all my heart now and forever.

Let me tell you a little about myself and how I got here :) I am the middle child of 3, raised on a farm in Kansas. If you have ever visited or lived in Kansas you may know that there are buffet's everywhere. Kentucky Fried Chicken has one, Taco Bell has one, and on and on and on. Hence 95% of my family is extremely over weight.

I left when I was 17 a senior in High School and moved to California with my mother. I have to say I have never been over weight per say, but I have had the mind of someone who is.

The obsession of my weight started in my teens. I was bulimic, took diet pills, exercised, stopped eating (for a day...I love food too much), etc. You see my point. They say what you think about, you bring about, well, I always worried about gaining weight... and guess what, and I did just that.

At age 24, I was getting married for the second time and weighed more than I ever had, except when I was pregnant. After coming home from my honeymoon my mother and I went to a weight doctor.

I love my mom, but she is the one who taught me how to play the yo-yo diet game. This doctor gave me the HCG injection, water pill, thyroid pill and a little black capsule that looked a lot like a speed pill called black beauty back in the day. I dropped 22 pounds in 6 weeks. This was my introduction to HCG, which was

22 years ago.

At the same time I was seeing this doctor I started a little job at a fitness facility. This is where I began my 15-year journey in the fitness industry as an aerobics instructor; that sure dates me; today they are called Group Exercise Instructors :) I loved teaching, it gave me the freedom to eat, basically, whatever I wanted and keep the weight off, as long as I worked out like a maniac.

In October of 2000 I met my current husband and my best friend. We married in 2002 and resided in Santa Clarita, California, where I had lived for 22 years. I knew everyone. I had taught in every fitness facility in the SC Valley. Every time I went shopping, got a cup of coffee, or ate at a restaurant, someone came up and said hello. Now this can surely feed ones ego and I had a big one to feed.

I wasn't aware of it until 2004 when Colin and I moved to Hermosa Beach. I had stopped teaching and moved to a community where I knew NO ONE. For 15 years I was used to working out with a group or with someone, riding my bike with someone, and running with someone...I think you've got the picture. I very rarely work out alone and yet I was now living in, a wonderful, beach community ALONE.

My 2 boys and 3 stepchildren lived in other cities. My husband ran our mortgage company in Santa Clarita, which was 35 miles away, from L.A. At the time it might as well have been 65 miles away. Needless to say he was gone 12 to 14 hours a day 5 to 6 days a week.

Within a few months I had an emotional breakdown. Going to the gym was not an option for me, I physically couldn't do it. After a year of counseling and acupuncture I was back on track, I successfully climbed over that mountain and was now able to focus on an older much bigger one, my weight.

Over that past year the pounds started to climb, and due to my lack of cardio and weight training, I couldn't say it was muscle, it wasn't! I started back on the "getting in shape", "Building Muscle", "Losing Weight" mountain.

I am sure by now you have read Colin's story, so you know how he and we had battled individually and/or collectively with our weight problem. We had tried everything from counting calories, interval training, endurance training, diet pills, diet books, pre-packaged foods, the lemon aid diet, the cabbage diet, etc. and nothing seemed to stick. We both were still playing yo-yo.

It was Thanksgiving 2007 and Colin and I were staying in Malibu for the holiday. We were alone and bored so we were watching the T.V. series "The Biggest Looser" They had a marathon going and we watch the whole season in one afternoon. It really inspired us to see the extreme transformations. Throughout the weekend we also watched Kevin Trudeau's infomercial about losing weight. We didn't know it then, but that moment would lead us to take the first steps towards our weight loss success and living our passion.

On Easter of 2008, we were celebrating with my oldest son and his family. I will never forget it because I made a chocolate Easter bunny cake, you know the one where you take 2 round cakes and cut ears and a bow tie out of one of the cakes, and the other is for the face.

Well I made the chocolate cake even better or worse depending how you look at it. I spread peanut butter on the entire cake and then layered milk chocolate frosting on top of that, not to mention the candy, which made the bunny's face, and the large Ghirardelli chocolate chips that out lined the bunny's bow tie and ears. We took a lot of pictures and ate like there was no tomorrow.

That cake was GONE by the time we left. Within a few days I saw a picture on My Space or one of those sites with me holding my grandson. Oh My Gosh!!! I looked swollen. I knew then that Colin and I had to do something and that day we ordered the Kevin Trudeau book, "Weight Loss Cure They Don't Want You to Know About".

By the time the book was delivered we were MORE than ready to start. With no expectation of what to do or what not to do, we were like two kids that just got a birthday present. You know it was the best present we had ever gotten ourselves. Colin did what Colin does and read the entire book.

I on the other hand read bits and pieces. I knew he would read it so I could expect him to know exactly what to do :) I read the first phase in the Kevin Trudeau book and started doing as much detoxing as I could afford, until Colin finished reading the entire book and we found a doctor, locally, that sold HCG.

Funny I KNEW that this would work when I found out it was HCG, because I had done it in my 20's. Colin on the other hand was skeptical, he felt like he had done almost everything and why would this be any different, but he jumped on the bandwagon with a positive mindset.

Looking back on it now I had NO idea how hard it was going to be based on my experience 20 years ago. When I had done it back then, I didn't have to count calories, prepare foods a certain way, not eat certain foods, only take in certain amount of calories, etc. because the doctor took care of any water weight I might have had, or any hunger that would creep up and boosted my metabolism. Hence back then; there was no diet to follow.

After reading the book, Colin got on the web and started searching for places to buy the HCG. The first one we inquired about was in Florida. The process, with this company, was too long and costly. He continued searching and finally found a doctor in Newport Beach, which was 35 miles from where we lived. Colin called to find out the process and the expense.

All we had to do was go get a blood test, wait for the results and then drive out to Newport Beach and get the HCG. Everything worked out well and within a week we had it, minus $1,200 out of our pockets. At this point of the game it was less than the company we found in Florida and we were determined.

It was the end of May when we started and within 46 days I dropped 25 pounds and Colin dropped 41. It worked, but let me tell you it was no walk in the park. Yes, we got daily instant gratification. This is probably why we continued the protocol past the 26 days.

Colin had a 10-year-old son, now 11, who lives with us and someone had to cook for him. Smelling the macaroni and cheese or chicken nuggets or spaghetti sauce or pancakes was painful and challenging. Thank God, within a matter of 3 weeks school would be out and he would be traveling to Ohio where he visits his mother for the summers. We love him, but preparing food, without tasting or taking a bite, on a daily basis was very hard to do.

Within those 45 days we also had a 4-day seminar in Los Angeles that started at 8:00 a.m. and ended at 11:00 p.m. How did we stay on track? We prepared our food the night before and put everything in an ice chest. While hundreds of people were eating lunch and dinner, we would go to our car and eat our food.

Then walk back to smell everyone else's lunch and dinner of hot dogs, burritos, hamburgers etc.

We would eat our apple or grapefruit during the breaks while everyone else was drinking cokes and eating muffins or cookies. I told you it was hard but we were two determined people and we had each other to support and encourage one another. That was one of the tools to our success.

Round two of the fourth time I've done the HCG Protocol. Why was it so much harder? One of the rewards we gave ourselves was a trip to Jamaica. Colin has an uncle who lives there and we went to visit and explore the island. Six weeks before leaving, we decided to do another round of HCG.

You know, get as thin as possible before vacation so you can eat and not feel as guilty, the operative word here is AS. Looking back on it now, I think when I reached MY goal weight the motivation to follow the protocol all the way through was gone. The first 3 to 4 days was good. I followed the diet to the tee. However, when that first hunger pain set in I added more protein or ate more Melba toast crackers. I justified this by saying "I look good enough". Needless to say I didn't make it more than 5 to 7 days before I fell off the wagon.

Our Jamaica trip was awesome. However, I did gain 5 pounds in 2 weeks. Colin and I had planned another trip to Mexico right before Christmas. I thought that I could take off the 5 pounds that I gained from Jamaica without the HCG. After all I did come from fitness background. I can drop 5 pounds within 3 months.... so I thought. I didn't drop the 5 pounds; in fact I gained another 3 to 4 pounds while in Mexico. Those all-inclusive resorts can sure get ya.

By March I decided that another round of HCG was needed. So there I go getting on the wagon again. This third round, I have to say, I stayed on track. In fact I completed the protocol eating raw. Nothing but fruits and raw vegetables. I felt great and lost 14 pounds. Eating raw was very interesting to me and it tasted great. I continued eating this way for another 5 months. I enjoyed the taste, but the preparation and the length of time to make a chip were too long for me. Well that is another story. Needless to say, I went back to my old eating habits.

Within a year I gained 15 pounds. I know I hear what you're saying, "I thought this protocol was supposed to re-set your hypothalamus gland and you would not gain the weight you lost back". It's about balance and since I am an emotional eater, my friend for the next year was sugar, flour, and processed foods. Did I eat cleaner than I ever had? Yes. But, obviously, my eating habits were out of balance. Maybe that is why it took me a year to put the weight back on.

This would be the fourth time taking HCG. I knew I would lose the 15 pounds I gained if I followed the protocol and now I knew what I had to do in order to keep the weight off, STAY CONSCIOUS! Why did I eat what I ate, when I ate it? It's all about choice.

Eating clean was not for just the 26 days or 43 days on HCG. It is a way of life. Will I not be able to eat another cookie or chip..? NO! It's all about balance and choice. I will NOT grow older without kicking and screaming ;) I KNOW what I put in my body is a direct effect of how my skin looks, the level of my energy, my mood, how my joints feel, etc. Every choice I make is either of love or fear. When I'm eating out of emotions, which is fear. When I put live foods, healthy foods in my body, it is love. I CHOOSE LOVE!

GOD   BLESS,
Jayne

Why & How HCG Body for Life Weight Loss System Works

If you want to lose 30 pounds in as little as thirty days then the HCG diet is what you have been looking for.

The HCG body for Life protocol works over and over again when most other popular, current diets fail. You don't need to spend a fortune in order to lose more weight than you ever did before.

When I decided to make the commitment to lose weight, I was told that I would need to wait 6 or 7 months in order to lose just 30 pounds. I don't know about you, but that seems like a very long time to wait.

I didn't want to wait that long so I kept looking for other alternatives.

The HCG diet is the one diet that I know, that promises incredible results and then DELIVERS results. Most diets make outrageous promises, but then deliver very little.

"The act of resisting something is the act of granting it life... the more you resist, the more you make it real? Whatever it is you are resisting."
Neale Donald Walsh

What Is The HCG Diet?

HCG stands for Human Chorionic Gonadotropin, the hormone produced by pregnant women in the early stages of pregnancy.

Research suggests a small, daily HCG injection (approx. 125 IU to 200 IU) may result in a weight loss of 1 to 2 lbs. per day, and often more, when accompanied by a VLCD (very low calorie diet of approximately 500 calories).

Burn the Fat and Reveal the Muscles

The thing that separates this diet from all others is that it is an extremely low calorie diet, but you are kept from being hungry. This is really the Holy Grail for people who want to lose weight. It is the HCG hormone that prevents the sensation of hunger.

Most people try to cut calories but they suffer from severe weight rebounds as they eventually give into the cravings. As such, most people who go on a diet actually end up being more overweight than when they started.

When you activate and introduce the HCG hormone, this will no longer be the case for you. This will ensure that you stay with the diet over the period of time needed to lose the weight you want.

How HCG Prevents Hunger Pains

HCG prevents hunger pains as it works on the Hypothalamus in the brain, which is what controls the brain. When HCG is not present, the Hypothalamus will send a trigger to the body and only burn structural fat and lean muscle tissue.

This is what results in short term weight loss, but the body will soon reach a plateau as it can no longer burn the structural fat and lean muscle.

When you use more HCG, your body will be told (by the hypothalamus) to burn more body fat than it usually will. Obviously, when your body burns more body fat, you reverse the process that leads to obesity.

HCG goes right to the fat stores that you want to get rid of, unlike most of the other diets out there. Many other diets actually lead your body to burn lean muscle tissue, which is the exact opposite of what you want (the more muscle you have, the more fat you will burn anyway).

HCG Targets the Root Cause of Weight Gain

As you can see, the HCG hormone targets the root cause of weight gain and obesity in a way that nothing else can. By burning the adipose tissue, you lose the right kind of weight and also maintain your lean muscle tissue (perfect for safe and healthy weight loss).

There are many other diets that use substances such as caffeine and herbal ephedra plus many other unknown ingredients. These things are used in order to raise the metabolism but they don't target the body fat solely.

There are often many dangerous side effects of using things of this nature, as they are not natural for the human body. In comparison, HCG is a natural hormone that the body needs in order to function correctly.

"Real integrity is doing the right thing,
knowing that nobody's going to know whether
you did it or not."
Oprah Winfrey

HCG Increases Your Energy by Burning Fat

Most people need carbohydrates for energy. And as you know, most carbohydrates lead to rapid increase in body fat. HCG is perfect for weight loss as it gives you the energy you need by burning the unwanted body fat.

When this happens, a signal is sent from the body to the brain, telling it that it has all the energy it needs. This therefore prevents hunger pains or food cravings from occurring.

HCG Had No Common Diet Side Effects

With most diets, the side effects soon become clear. The low calories that people consume soon lead to headaches, lack of energy, apathy, and sometimes-psychological issues.

As HCG tells the brains that the body has enough energy, these side effects are overcome. If you need more energy, then your body will just burn more adipose tissue. As such your body will get all the nutrients it needs without going into starvation mode.

Once again, HCG is natural and works with the body – not against it.

I have included a clinical study that was printed in the American

Journal of Clinical Nutrition. You will see that scientific findings back up what you have just read (and my own personal experience).

HCG Weight Loss Clinical Study

American Journal of Clinical Nutrition
www.ajcn.org and the American Society of Bariatric Physicians Research Council, 333 West Hampden Avenue, Englewood, Colorado 80110

Effect of human chorionic gonadotropin on weight loss, hunger, and feeling of well-being

Authored by: W. L. Asher, MD and Harold W. Harper, MD

Twenty female patients on 500- to 550- kcal diets receiving daily injections of 125 IU of human chorionic gonadotropin (HCG) were compared with 20 female patients on 500- to 550-kcal diets receiving placebo injections.

Patients in both groups were instructed to return for daily injections 6 days each week for a total of 36 injections (unless desired weight was achieved prior to this).

The HCG group lost significantly more mean weight, had a significantly greater mean weight loss per injection, and lost a significantly greater mean percentage of their starting weight. The percentage of affirmative daily patient responses indicating "little or no hunger" and "feeling good to excellent" was significantly greater in the HCG group than in the placebo group.

Additional investigation of the influence of HCG on weight loss, hunger, and well-being seems indicated.

American Journal of Clinical Nutrition, Volume 26, 211-218, Copyright © 1973 by the American Society for Clinical Nutrition, Inc.

"Joy is what happens when we allow ourselves to recognize how good things really are."
                                                    Marianne Williamson

The Need for Increased Protein Portions

I discovered in my personal experiment that the original protein portions recommended by Dr. Simeons were too low to sustain optimal fat loss. The 3.5 oz. or 100 grams of lean protein may have been sufficient in the 1950's 60' and even the 70's may have been sufficient, however today in 2010, this is no longer the case.

In the example below, you will get a better idea of what I am referring to.

I found this list to be very helpful when I was looking for the some answer...

Fish:
- White Fish - (3.5 oz.) avg 98 cal
- Cod (3.5 oz.) - 83 cal
- Crab meat (3.5 oz.) - 100 cal
- Flounder (3.5 oz.) - 90 cal
- Haddock (3.5 oz.) - 88 cal
- Halibut (3.5 oz.) - 110 cal
- Lobster (3.5 oz.) - 98 cal
- Red snapper (3.5 oz.) - 110 cal
- Shrimp (3.5 oz.) - 110 cal
- Tilapia (3.5 oz.) - 94 cal

Beef:
- Very lean beef (3.5 oz.) (avg 152 cal)
- Eye of round (3.5 oz.) - 160 cal
- Top sirloin steak (3.5 oz.) - 130 cal
- Top round steak (3.5 oz.) - 166 cal
- Bottom round steak (3.5 oz.) - 154 cal

Chicken:
- Chicken breast, no skin (3.5 oz.) - 87 cal

Veal:
- Veal (3.5 oz.) (avg 114 cal)
- Veal, sirloin (3.5 oz.) - 110 cal
- Veal, loin chop (3.5 oz.) - 117 cal

Vegetables:
- Asparagus (3.5 oz.) - 20 cal
- Asparagus (2" tip) - 1 cal
- Asparagus (small spear) - 2 cal
- Asparagus (medium spear) - 3 cal
- Asparagus (large spear) - 4 cal
- Celery (3.5 oz.) - 15 cal
- Celery (medium stalk) - 6 cal
- Cabbage (3.5 oz.) - 24 cal
- Cabbage (1 cup shredded) - 17 cal
- Cucumber (3.5 oz.) - 12 cal
- Cucumber (small) - 19 cal
- Cucumber (medium) - 24 cal
- Cucumber (large) - 34 cal each

- Cucumber (English long) - 60 cal
- Onions cooked (1 cup) – 92 cal
- Swiss chard, cooked (1 cup) – 35 cal
- Lettuce, all varieties (3.5 oz.) - 20 cal
- Lettuce, all varieties (1 cup) - 8 cal
- Lettuce, all varieties (small head) - 32 cal
- Red radishes (3.5 oz.) - 12 cal
- Red radishes (one medium) - 1 cal
- Salad (3.5 oz.) - 15 cal
- Spinach, raw (3.5 oz.) - 20 cal
- Spinach, raw (1 cup) - 7 cal
- Spinach, frozen (3.5 oz.) - 23 cal
- Spinach, frozen (1 cup) - 41 cal
- Spinach, cooked (3.5 oz.) - 31 cal
- Spinach, cooked (1 cup) - 48 cal
- Tomato (3.5 oz.) - 20 cal
- Tomato (cherry) - 3 cal
- Tomato (plumb) - 11 cal
- Tomato (small) - 16 cal
- Tomato (medium) - 22 cal
- Tomato (large) - 33 cal
- Fennel (1 cup) – 27 cal

Fruit
- Apple (small) - 55 cal
- Apple (medium) - 72 cal
- Apple (large) - 110 cal
- Orange (navel) - 69 cal

- 12 large strawberries - 72 cal
- 20 medium strawberries - 80 cal
- Pink Grapefruit (California) - 92 cal
- Pink Grapefruit (Florida) - 74 cal

Grain
- One bread stick (grissini) - 15 cal
- One Melba toast - 12 cal

When you take for example, White Fish - (3.5 oz.) 98 calories add in some Asparagus (3.5 oz.) - 20 calories then add in your fruit of one Apple (medium) - 72 calories and one bread stick (grissini) - 15 calories, your first meal of the day ads up to (205) calories.

Then let's put your second meal together using Dr. Simeon's recommendations. We'll start with a Chicken breast, no skin (3.5 oz.) - 87 calories, add in some Cucumber slices (large) - 34 calories and 6 large strawberries - 36 calories and One Melba toast - 12 calories, your second meal would add up to 169 calories. Your total calorie intake for the day would be (374 **calories)** a diet this low in calories regardless of having HCG in your body would trigger the starvation response in your body and force your metabolism to shut down, or switch from burning body fat to using lean muscle tissue for fuel. In order to correct this flaw in the original protocol, we have made a few strategic adjustments to the protein portions and created a meal plan that provides the body the necessary nutrients, and daily calorie intake to increase fat loss and help you build a new lean sexier body.

Your daily Intake at a glance
½ A GALLON MINIMUM OF FLUIDS
2-3 FRUIT SERVINGS
2-3 PROTEIN SERVINGS
Egg whites are included as 1 of the 3 proteins
2 VEGETABLE SERVINGS
1-2 SMALL SALADS
DO NOT GO ABOVE 750 CALORIES PER DAY!

HCG BODY FOR LIFE ESSENTIALS
- **Braggs Organic Apple Cider Vinegar**
- **Braggs All Natural Liquid Aminos**
- **Stevia Natural Sweetener**
- **All Natural Sea Salt**
- **Food Scale**
- **Accurate Weight Scale**
- **Tape Measure**
- **Organic Coconut Oil**
- **MTC Oil or Mineral Oil**

PHASE TWO (2) MENU GUIDE

DRINK
Bottled or filtered water (no tap water)
Mineral water
Black coffee
1 to 2-tbsp/day Lucerne sugar free/fat free (Not Recommended: Only for the coffee desperate)
French Vanilla coffee creamer
Unsweetened organic soy milk (2 tbsp/day)
Herbal teas (any tea bag assortment)
No dairy products (except for egg whites)
No alcoholic beverages
No sodas, no diet drinks, no protein shakes, no crystal light

BREAKFAST
Drink plenty of tea and bottled or filtered water. You may have 1 fruit for breakfast and 3 egg <u>whites</u>. (ONLY)

LUNCH and DINNER

Are exactly the same food choices (1 protein 1 fruit, 1 to 2 vegetable and 1 small salad)

PROTEIN

- Choose 1 of the following proteins for lunch and dinner.

- ☐ **Red Meat**- Filet mignon (the leanest), top sirloin, organic grass fed beef, buffalo, veal (about 180 calories) Only Ground TURKEY.
- ☐ **Chicken**- Organic preferred or antibiotic free breast of chicken (skinless), white meat only (about 223 calories)
- ☐ **White Fish ONLY**- Examples include: Tilapia, cod, halibut, sea bass, sole, flounder, grouper, canned white tuna (low sodium), shrimp, lobster, scallops and crab. Any white fish is acceptable. No Salmon….it is orange!
- ☐ Eat approximately (3.5 to 6 oz. See Food Chart) of protein (about the size of the palm of your hand)
- ☐ Grill or bake your proteins. Do not use any cooking oils, butter or margarine. **(only 1tsp organic extra virgin coconut oil)**

(See Acceptable Condiments list on the next page and our HCG Body for Life Cookbook)

VEGETABLE –
- ☐ 2 servings per day.
- ☐ Choose 1 serving of **green** vegetables for lunch and dinner.
- ☐ Eat 1 cup of cooked green vegetables.

These can be eaten raw, steamed, grilled (with 1tsp organic coconut oil) per serving.
If it <u>isn't green</u>, do not eat it.

HCG BODY FOR LIFE PROTEIN CHART

Food Item	Cal Per Oz	Oz Eaten	Total Cal
Apple	5	4	60
½ Grapefruit	9	6.6	59.4
Strawberries	9	6.6	59.4
Asparagus	6	6.7	40.2
Beet Greens	6	6.7	40.2

Broccoli	10	3.2	30
Cabbage	7	5.7	39.9
Celery	4	10	40
Chard	7	5.7	39.9
Chicory	7	5.7	39.9
Cucumber	3	13	39
Fennel	9	4.5	40.5
Romaine Let	5	8	40
Iceberg Let	4	10	40
Onion, bulb	12	3.3	39.6
Onion, green	9	4.5	40.5
Radish	5	8	40
Spinach	7	5.7	39.9
Tomato	5	8	40

1-tsp Coconut Oil   39

PROTEIN CHOICES

Chicken	31	4.85	150.35
King Crab	24	6.25	150
Founder/Sole	26	5.8	150.8
Alaskan Sea Bass	28	5.8	150.8
Tilapia	27	5.55	149.85
Cod	23	6.5	149
Halibut	31	4.85	150.35
Ground Turkey 93%	41	3.66	150.06
Ground Turkey 99%	30	5	150
Hamburger 95%	38	3.95	150.1
Prawn	30	5	150
Steak, sirloin	53	2.83	149.99
Scallops	25	6	150
Shrimp, shelled	30	5	150
Lobster	26	5.8	150.8
1 Egg & 4 Whites	15	10	150

Examples Meal One Below:
4.85 oz. Chicken breast = 150.00
Spinach, cooked (1 cup) – 48
Asparagus - 20 calories sautéed in 1 tsp. coconut oil – 39 calories
Apple (medium) - 72 calories

Total calories for meal one = 309 calories.

SALAD
(1-2 small per day)
You may eat a salad with your meal or in between your meals. Use any green leaf lettuce, tomato, fresh onion, cucumber and celery with Bragg's or generic equivalent with 1tsp coconut oil- Organic Apple Cider Raw Unfiltered Vinegar that contains NO FAT. Lemon juice may also be used as a salad dressing.

FRUIT
(2 1/2-3 per day-organic preferred)

Eat 2-3 fruits per day with your meals or in between.
1 grapefruit large
1 apple small, medium, or large
1 handful of strawberries
*** *There are no fruit substitutes****
*** *No lima beans or peas* ***

Do not to eat the <u>same protein, vegetable or fruit combinations</u> twice in the same day if possible. Metabolic activity may increase by following this concept suggested by Dr. Simeons.

The Mental Aspect of The Diet

I am so excited for you to begin your journey. I cannot truly express in words what it feels like to have the body I have today, and feel the way I do about myself.

Regaining my self-esteem and overall good health was absolutely priceless. I want you to know up front that I was not being paid in any way to share this information with you when writing my blogs, and doing my radio show.

I have several other businesses and activities that I do that bring me joy and prosperity. Sharing this information has become a passion of mine as well. I decided to create a website because so many people ask me on a daily basis, how I transformed my body, and became prescription free from high blood pressure medications, and turned back the clock on what we call our family curse of Diabetes.

My grandparents, father and mother are all deceased from either Diabetes related illnesses or heart failure.

At age 49, I am as healthy today as I was when I was twenty-five years old. This diet protocol will take dedication from you, and support from your direct family members.

If you are married or have a significant other, get them on the same page or on this protocol, or make sure they are willing to support you while you complete the one or two 26, 43, or 60 day cycles.

Motivation

I've always been entertained from watching squirrels but I never thought I would feel motivated from watching squirrels.

http://www.youtube.com/watch?v=1jByfWOLmjo&feature=player_embedded
Audio link==➜ Download audio:
http://tinyurl.com/DontBeATryBaby

In fact, this baby squirrel was so inspiring that I actually watched the video over and over again so I could take some notes. Here is how it relates to motivation and staying on track with your weight loss goal:

If you want to achieve any goal, your first step is to declare it. These squirrels started their day with one goal in mind – get the baby squirrel to the top of the wall!

They took 100% responsibility for creating the goal and did not stop until the baby squirrel made it to the top of the wall! As far as setting goals and actually achieving them, squirrels have a major advantage over humans.

The words "hopefully," "can't," "maybe" — and the ultimate death trap for goals — "try" do not exist for squirrels! At one point in our lives, they didn't exist for us either.

When we were children, we had an amazing ability to dream. What does your dream body look like? I saw mine when LL Cool J, lifted his shirt in the movie "SWAT".

"We change the world not by what we say or do, but as a consequence of what we have become." David R. Hawkins

I was like "Daaaaahum, now that's what I'm talking about". That became my goal, and I didn't fall too short of that.

As a child, you never said "I'm going to try to be a (insert your dream body idol from childhood here)." You said "I'm going to look just like a _____!"

Today I challenge you to forget what everyone like your parents and teachers, your friends, family members and colleagues said about "being realistic" or "getting your head out of the clouds..." Forget your goals of having just an ok physique this summer!

Start dreaming big again TODAY!

Believe it or not, it just takes a little more effort to achieve a great body than it does to just lose a little weight.

Surround Yourself with Greatness

As these adorable squirrels proved, it's a fact of life that people tend to mimic what they see around them. The baby squirrel watched the big squirrel dart up and down the seemingly 'HUGE' wall like it was nothing.
After a little encouragement from the big squirrel, the baby squirrel was eventually able to dig up the courage to make it to the top! The same thing goes for you... If you surround yourself with successful healthy, fit people, then you'll want to fit in and be fit and healthy, too!

What do you think happens when people surround themselves with negative, unhealthy, out of shape people with small dreams and low self-esteem?

They forget their big dreams and start accepting that 'realistic' body and life everyone kept telling them about.

"When the pupil is ready, the teacher will appear."   *Unknown*

Audio link==➔ Download audio:
http://tinyurl.com/hcgdietpreparementally

Previous Failed Diet Attempts

Most of the people that read this book have probably tried many diet plans before. If you read my story then you know that I tried everything before I gave the HCG diet a chance.

You might be worried that you will never be able to complete the HCG diet, or may have some fear of failure again. This is quite normal, but you need to go ahead and overcome these limiting beliefs.

Learning to eat healthy is a work in progress and just like any skill, it takes time to master.

We are often our own worst enemy when it comes to completing a diet plan successfully. It's easy to sabotage yourself by storing the wrong food in the house or forgetting to plan or in some cases, prepare your meals ahead of time to limit the possibilities of eating the wrong foods in desperation.

You may feel that you "deserve it" because you stuck to the diet all week. Or maybe you "deserve it" because you had a bad day.

The key, of course, is to plan ahead, and keep healthy food around you at all times, stay focused and committed to keeping the end goal in mind.

Here is a great tactic to stay on track:

What is your Purpose?

What is your "Why"?   Ask yourself why you are doing this protocol?

These questions are very important. Are you sick of being overweight? Are you tired of buying clothes that look great in the store window but not quite as good in your size?

Do you want this summer to be the one that you feel comfortable in your swimming suit? Are you just about ready to get married and want to have the body that you've always dreamed about? Are you just plain tired of being sick and tired?

Whatever your reason is, you need to keep it in the forefront of "Your Mind".

Picture yourself and feel the feelings of how you'll feel when you achieve your goal. Plan a way to reward yourself (something that is non-food related).

Most importantly, if you happen to "Back Slide" then acknowledge your mistake, and seek to understand the circumstances that caused you to make these choices and create strategies to prevent it from happening again. The worst thing you can do is to blame it on the diet, the product or your individual circumstance. No excuses!

"When you judge another, you do not define them, you define yourself" By Wayne Dyer

1. ➔ http://tinyurl.com/meditaion

2. ➔ http://tinyurl.com/excusbegone

Stress

I think one really important thing you could do for yourself is alleviating your stress. This is very important when trying to lose weight.

For example, something happens, you get in a fight with somebody or something happens at work, or you get run off the road and all of a sudden the first thing you want to do is to eat something.

I've got to tell you that this protocol will expose your weaknesses. It'll expose your emotional triggers and you want to know why?

Suddenly you're not really physically hungry but you're mentally hungry because you want to do something to feed that anxiety inside of you.

I really believe that listening to something calm and meditative actually works wonders on the diet. And for me, visualization was a huge process of transforming my body -- not just losing weight but transforming my body.
If you have seen my before and after pictures, I didn't look like I was in the greatest shape. It wasn't like I had any peer pressure to lose weight other than the fact that I knew that my personal image of myself wasn't great. I wasn't feeling real good about it.

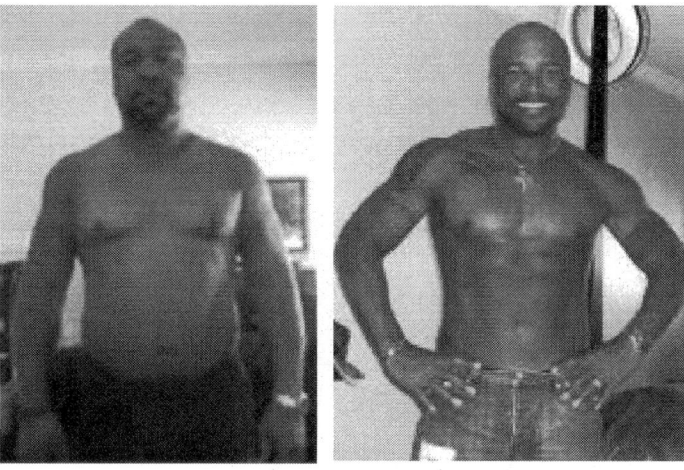

Figure 1 – BEFORE   Figure 2 – AFTER

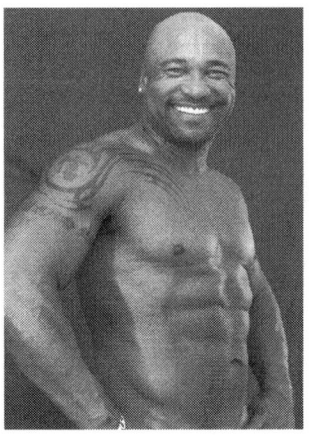

Figure 3 – TODAY

I'm now in a position where I have younger guys who want to work out with me and they think I'm a body builder even though I'm not.

The point is: to be seen in that class is a huge leap from where I was at, from being just a big guy to "Hey where do you live? You're a body builder?"

It just feels really good. This is an opportunity to visualize the transformation you want. And make no mistake, what you think about, you bring about.

Believe it or not, you brought about being overweight, by thinking about how much you did not want to be fat or overweight by focusing on it day in and day out. Therefore, it's kind of like reversing that thought process and focusing your thinking on creating a positive body image in order to get the body that you've always wanted.

I recommend a Wayne Dyer product. Either "Meditation for Manifestation" or his "Excuses Begone!"

"Excuses Begone!" is a powerful CD series that talks about all the Mickey Mouse excuses we give ourselves to thwart our destiny, to get in the way of our own progress and in the way of our own destiny. By adding this in with the advanced HCG weight loss system, which works 100% of the time as long as you follow it, you're going to have guaranteed success and a guaranteed transformation not just a body transformation but also a life transformation.

There's something that clicks inside of you when you realize you've accomplished something, when you've accomplished something that has beaten you most of your life. Most of the people that I've talked to have either been athletes and got injured or suddenly had their life changed (they got married) and their bodies changed. Either way, they didn't pay attention and the body fat got the best of them.

And it's discouraging, it's frustrating and I'm sure there are many of you that are skeptical that this is going to even work for you too.

"Realize deeply that the present moment is all you ever have. Make the Now the primary focus of your life"   - Eckhart Tolle

You want to be able to get your mind right and get your mindset around the fact that this is absolutely going to happen, it's absolutely possible, and that you can transform your body in record time.

I'm talking about in 26 days or 43 days. The payoff is the weight you have to lose. But the progress you make in that period of time is worth it.

It's almost a mental game you play with yourself because of how much you're going to weigh. I might drop a pound, I might drop 2 pounds and it motivates you every single day not to mess up because you know tomorrow you're going to get a reward.

You need to have some sort of peace of mind, body and soul meditation or someplace, something that can always keep affirming that you're on the right path and that you're going to reach your goal. I think it is absolutely paramount for success.

This is not a diet that you try. You just do it. Whatever has gotten in your way in the past, doesn't have to get in your way this time.

The HCG Protocol Explained

This protocol started when the late British Physician, Dr. A. T. W. Simeons discovered the HCG weight loss protocol over fifty years ago. He devoted years to research and treated thousands of patients suffering from obesity.

During this time, Simeons noticed several important factors including the lack of symptoms one would expect from a patient on a very low calorie diet. For example, his patients had no headaches, hunger pains, weakness, or irritability as long as the low calorie diet was combined with HCG Shots.

Tens of thousands of people used this simple, inexpensive, safe treatment and achieved substantial and permanent weight loss.

The main problems that overweight people deal with are massive, intense, constant physical hunger; food cravings and uncontrollable urges to eat when not hungry; low metabolism; and a high amount of fat stored in stubborn secure problem areas such as the hips, thighs, buttocks, and waist.

The HCG weight loss plan helps with all of these problems along with the HCG Injections.

HCG Diet Original vs. New Advanced HCG Weight Loss System Explained

The History of HCG

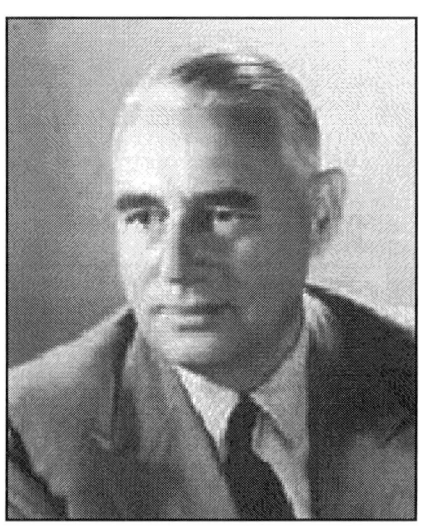

In 1967, Dr. Albert T. Simeons, a British-born physician, became the foundation of a weight loss program that used a medication called HCG (Human Chorionic Gonadotropin), a hormone produced when a woman becomes pregnant.

Dr. Simeons discovered that if HCG can utilize the body's own fat reserves for nutrition to the baby in periods of deprivation, then a small amount administered daily in non-pregnant women and men may assist in weight loss.

It is believed that HCG may assist in the removal of stored fat by liquefying the fat cell contents, utilizing it as energy and then eliminating it through the body's own elimination process.

Under the direction of a licensed physician, the patient would receive an injection of the HCG medication daily and administered into the fatty tissue (belly area preferred) for a period of 23-40 days.

Women on average may lose 25-40 pounds and men may lose 35-47 lbs. in a 3-6 week period.

Dr. Simeons created a research manual, "Pounds and Inches" that focused on the use of HCG as a weight loss solution and found that HCG alone will not cause weight loss.

"Walk away from what doesn't work. Work towards what does."

However, if used in combination with a specific low calorie diet, combined with some exercise, significant weight loss may possibly occur.

By the 1970's HCG was the most widespread obesity medication administered in the United States. In 1976, the FTC ordered that Dr. Simeons and his associated group, stop claiming that their HCG based programs were safe, effective, and/or approved by the FDA for weight-control.

Although the order did not stop the clinics from using HCG, it required that patients who wanted the treatment be informed in writing that: "HCG has not been demonstrated to be an effective adjunctive therapy in the treatment of obesity. There is no substantial evidence that it increases weight loss beyond that resulting from caloric restriction, that it causes a more attractive "normal" distribution of fat or that it decreases the hunger and discomfort associated with calorie-restricted diets."

Since then, there have been thousands of success stories using HCG for weight loss including a book that sold over 4 million copies that reached the New York Times Best Sellers List.

HCG has not been approved by the FDA as a weight loss medication and using HCG alone may not guarantee weight loss results. HCG is only a small part of a specialized weight management and lifestyle program.

In order to achieve success, the entire program must be followed.

"Happiness cannot be traveled to, owned, earned, worn or consumed. Happiness is the spiritual experience of living every minute with love, grace and gratitude. " Denis Waitley

The Advanced HCG Diet Protocol Comparison Chart

HCG BFL Weight Loss Protocol	Original Dr. Simeons Protocol

1) 550 -750 calories daily	1) 500 calories daily
2) Eat breakfast	2) No breakfast, only tea
3) Effectively is an LCD; is safer than the original	3) Effectively a VLCD mandating closer supervision
4) More selection of green vegetables	4) Limited on vegetable intake
5) HCG is infused with methyl B12 or B12 injections	5) No B12
6) Multi-vitamin/minerals highly suggested	6) No vitamins except calcium
7) Take all medications prescribed by own MD	7) Prefers to stop all medications
8) Oral HCG drops available equally as effective. No discomfort.	8) Dr. Simeons gave his patients only intramuscular injections that were sometimes painful.
9) Self-administered Sub cutaneous injections or Sublingual HCG drops	9) Patients had to see Dr. Simeons every day for injections.

method	
10) HCG available in sublingual form	10) No sublingual form
11) Detailed HCG Diet Weight loss Book that is an exceptional educational tool.	11) Hard to understand pamphlet "Pounds and Inches" written 50 years ago, very confusing to most.
12) Cookbook for Phase 2 and Phase 3 meals with shopping list	12) Very ambiguous list of food to prepare
13) Exercise encouraged for maximum fat loss including HIIT (High Intensity Interval Training) video series workout	13) Popular perception (although wrong) is that exercise is either discouraged or not required.

Medication

People who are considering the HCG diet often wonder about the best way to get HCG into their bodies quickly and effectively.

Most believe that HCG shots are the best way to do this, while others find that sub-lingual HCG drops work best for them. Others swear by HCG pills. Which of these is the most effective, and which one should you utilize?

Out of the three main ways to take HCG, pills are the least effective. There is nothing inherently wrong with HCG when taken in tablet form, except that it probably won't work well for you assuming that it works at all.

In most types of hormone therapy, it's best to avoid absorption through the digestive tract, because the digestive enzymes in the stomach will destroy them very quickly. Hormones are a form of protein, chemically not very different than a piece of meat or fish.

According to a 1977 study in the Journal of the American Medical Association, HCG pills lose between 40% and 90% of their active ingredient when they go through the stomach. You may get some benefit, but it will be greatly reduced.

In addition, HCG pills are expensive – and you may wind up having to take them for a much longer period of time before they have any effect.

About Injections

HCG injections are a highly effective way to get the medication into your system.

However, in the past, these require a prescription from a physician, and many general practitioners will not write such prescriptions – if only because they don't know a great deal about HCG as a weight loss treatment.

However, with the Internet, you can now purchase HCG without a prescription for a fraction of the costs you would spend at these HCG weight loss clinics that offers this option.

HCG Shots can be uncomfortable for some people, but the upside is that you only need to take one shot a day with a very tiny insulin needle. This is the most convenient way to take HCG and offers the lowest overall, out of pocket HCG expense.

The Advantage of HCG Drops

When placed under the tongue (this is another way of taking Sub-Lingual or HCG drops). HCG gets into the bloodstream within a few minutes. In addition, HCG drops are also inexpensive, and you can order through the same trusted sites outlined on our website and by mixing the Sub-lingual HCG you know you are getting the real HCG and not a placebo.

Many websites are offering homeopathic HCG. To my understanding, this is not actually HCG at all. The best part is that HCG drops are very easy to use and can be taken right away, however, they must be taken several times a day.

Injection Procedure

Video Link==➔ http://www.youtube.com/watch?v=R4sQwZiSiXk

How to mix 5000IU'S of HCG for 200IU Daily Injection

Take out the supplies you will need in order to follow these instructions:

1. 30ml bacteriostatic water
2. 10ml clear bottle
3. HCG vial
4. 5ml syringe and mixing needle alcohol pads

First, you need to put together the supplies listed above in order to complete the mixing instruction.

You need to have a 10-ml clear mixing bottle. This is your mixing bottle. You need your bacteriostatic water and you are going to have a mixing needle with 5ml's or larger.

You will also have alcohol swabs to use to clean the surfaces of all of your supplies. Use it to clean the surfaces of the ampoules and mixing bottle and bacteriostatic bottles.

You can remove the sodium chloride that comes with your HCG, because you don't really need it, you can take it out and put it to the side.

Your HCG usually comes with a little red or blue cap on it, or it may also come in ampoules. Snap the lid off and you will see a white substance, or little white pellet in there and that is your HCG.

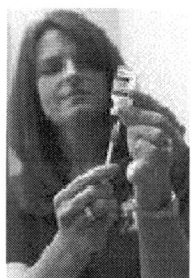

Genuine HCG comes usually in this powder form. Sometimes the supplier will send you a premixed liquid form, which is mixed with a 1-ml solution also inside this size bottle, but it is still in the powder form to begin with. Just so you know this is what it looks like.

Overview-1 ml of bacteriostatic water; I'm going to inject it into this small HCG bottle to dilute the pellet of HCG then extract the 1ml mixed solution of HCG from the small vial and add it to the 10ml clear vial.

Then you're going to add 4 more ml of bacteriostatic water. 5000IU's of HCG to 5 ml of bacteriostatic water, 5 to 5, very is easy to remember.

Here are the steps that you need to take:

1. First, clean the surfaces all of your mixing bottles, right now. Let's go ahead and just make sure that everything is sterile. By cleaning all these areas to begin with you'll know that you are using a clean and sterile surface.

2. This would be a brand new needle, go ahead and use that. You are going to take 1 ml of water from the BAC bottle, and add it to your HCG vial. Gently swirls your mixture to make sure all of your HCG has been dissolved. You're going to pressurizes this bottle and make it easier to extract the HCG from the vial and fill your syringe.

3. Extract all the HCG as much as you can, try and get every drop of it from this bottle. If there is a little teeny bit of liquid still in there it's not a big deal. Take that solution and put it into your big 10-ml clear bottle. This is the beginning of your mixture.

    Then you'll extract 4 more ml from your bacteriostatic water bottle. Pressurize the bacteriostatic water bottle by injecting 5ml of air into the bottle.

4. Fill your 5ml needle all the way up to the 4-ml mark. Put the 4 ml BAC water into your 10 ml mixing bottle that now contains your HCG mixture. You should now have a total of 5ml of HCG.

FINISHED PRODUCT-5000IU's plus 5ml's bacteriostatic water = dosage of 200IUs of HCG daily.

This should last you about 23 days which is the right amount of shots for the 26-day cycle. Duplicate this process on your 23-day to continue through the 43-day protocol.

You can also watch the video at www.HCGBodyforLife.com

A radiant and happy life will open up just by having radiant and happy thoughts ~ Ryuho Okawa

How Much HCG to Inject and How to Fill the Syringe

Video Link➔ http://www.youtube.com/watch?v=JOVpKKPsOBw

I've had a lot of e-mails about how much HCG to actually put in the syringe and people aren't sure what size of syringes that they're getting.

If you're getting the insulin needles (which are what I recommend, because it's not as long) or if you choose larger needles, I'd still be able to show you how much HCG to put into your syringe.

Now go over to the fridge where you store your HCG and let's see if I can help you figure that out.

Keep the HCG refrigerated at all times so you can make sure it stays fresh. You should fill your syringe to the .20 mark and inject this amount daily. (This is approximately 200 IU's).

This amount seems to work best for most dieters.

With that said, you always want to keep this clean and sterile. If you're touching it a lot, make sure you put alcohol swab on there and use the needle coming out of the package. When injecting, put the needle into the bottle (in the center) and then usually what I do is to inject some here and there so I can get the HCG out.

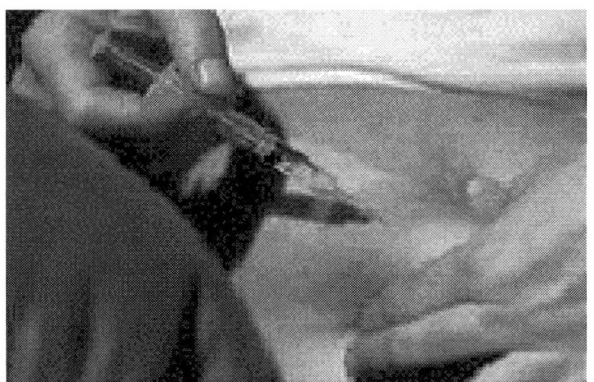

I usually overfill it (over 2) and then I push back into it at a downward angle to the .20 units mark. That gets the air bubbles out and you have your .20 units or **20** mark. You may also have needles that say 50 units instead of 100 units, but it's still going to be the same number, the 20. And that's 200 IU's.

Put that back on and you're ready to go. If you happen to have a larger needle for some reason and you'll see here that this one has 3ml but it's larger, you're still going be on the no. 2nd hash line of the large syringe line on this syringe.

For further clarification, simply copy and paste the video website link above in you Internet browser to watch an easy to follow instructional video.

HCG BFL Diet Phases

Mastering HCG BFL Diet – Gorging Phase 1

Audio link==➔ Download audio: http://tinyurl.com/hcgdietphase1

Phase 1 is called the gorge phase of the diet. It's a very interesting psychological thing that happens to people when they realize that you're now given permission for the first two days while you're on shots to eat anything and everything as fattening as you can eat to your heart's content for 48 hours. Many people fail to take this phase seriously.

This phase sets the stage for how much weight and how quickly you'll lose weight for the rest of the protocol. Messing up in Phase 1 or not completing it or not doing it true to protocol will definitely hinder your overall weight loss.

It's very important that you actually celebrate all the things you think you're going to possibly miss over the next 3 weeks to 6 weeks and indulge yourself to your heart's content.

Usually, the feeling you have at the end of day 2 is you are so sick of food, you are so sick of sugar, and sick of looking at food that you are just begging to get on something that's going to be clean eating and a sensible diet.

I think it was brilliant because there's a reason for it; you've got to gain before you can lose. I basically created a visual and I hope it helps you. Think of how HCG needs to find where you store your food, and where you store your fat in your body.

As you're eating fat while on HCG, you're basically leaving a trail to all the parts in your body where your body is storing your fat. So, when you finally go to the third day and you go to your very low calorie diet, the HCG knows exactly where to go to attack to release that fat.

Think of it that you are trying to signal HCG in your body to go to all the places in your body to release the fat. That's why Phase 1, the gorge phase, is so important.

You must consume as many different fattening foods that you can. Eat the foods that you love, get it out of your system because psychologically, you'll be ready to get a clean diet to have lower food content and better quality of food.

Mastering HCG Diet - Phase 2

Audio link==➔ Download audio: http://tinyurl.com/hcgdietbasics

Phase 2 is the very low calorie diet. Now, what it consists of is specific lean proteins and specific vegetables that work together synergistically in the body to help release the fat and also give you all the nutrients you need.

It is really important that you don't try to create your own diet. Believe it or not, this diet is not very forgiving at all. Sometimes even the slightest deviation from the diet can cause you not to lose weight, to stall.

And whenever you decide to cheat on this diet, you will stall your weight anywhere between three to five days and some people have done it for longer than that. Having personally been stuck at the "no weight loss stage" for up to three to five days, I know it is not very forgiving.

I think it's very simple to follow this diet. It's in black and white. The best thing to do is to print it out and keep it with you. If you don't see it on there, the answer is no. I have so many people ask me, "What about this food?" No. "What about that?" No.

If it's not on the diet and it's not in black and white, it's not allowed. This advanced HCG weight loss system has a 100% success rate if you just simply follow it. It's similar to building a table for my kids. You get the construction plan, you take out the pieces, you follow the instructions, you put all the bolts in there, make sure all the bolts and screws are all there so that the table would be sound and steady; very simple.

With that said, let's focus on the shopping list, and the things you need to put together.

- HCG
- Either an HCG mixing kit - either sublingual, which is oral drops, or injections
- **Buy HCG and HCG Mixing Kits Here ==→** http://hcgbodyforlife.com/

Those are the two keys of the puzzle.

Video Link ==→
http://www.youtube.com/watch?v=SzG61otOV3M

The other thing that makes it possible for you to complete the diet with ease is a body weight scale. The scale is going to be your barometer of your progress for the rest of your life.

You need to have a scale because you need to know when you're losing weight and when you're not. Because if you don't lose on any given day, it is an indicator that something went wrong the day previously.

Maybe you ate something, you did something, you shifted up something, you took too much of a portion, or you snuck a cough drop and you didn't realize what you were doing.

You also need to have a digital food scale. You need to weigh your portions. This is actually a habit that's going to save you for the rest of your life. Portion control is the key to maintaining our bodies.

We usually cook too much, eat too much, regret it later, and sit back and feel uncomfortable and go, "Oh, I shouldn't have eaten that much." Well guess what? If you only cook what you need, only prepare the foods you need which is what this diet teaches you to do; you will only eat what you need to be comfortable and to feed yourself.

The scale is important because you have to weigh everything. And when I mean everything, this does not include your vegetables per serving.

A handful of this and handful of that control vegetables. Your handful for your body is your portioned control. But when it comes to proteins, meat and fish, you need to measure them.

You can't have more than the correct portions for each protein source (See food chart pdf) Measure out the exact amount of the right ounces for the proteins on any given meal. The scale is absolutely essential.

Now some of the things that they never talked about in the original protocol that have been very beneficial are supplements. I'm going to go over some things that make your life a lot easier.

Organic extra virgin coconut oil

Kevin Trudeau introduced this in his revised version of the HCG Diet. It's a lifesaver because it covers a couple of different things. No. 1, you can't use any oils on this diet on the original protocol except for this organic coconut oil.

Organic coconut oil has a great deal of benefit to you that I didn't know about until I started doing this protocol. It actually promotes weight loss. It controls your cholesterol. It helps you with your immune system, proper digestion, your metabolism; it relieves kidney problems, and helps with heart disease and blood pressure.

Not only does it taste good with your food, you can actually cook your food in one teaspoon per serving. Let's say if you're cooking for one person, one teaspoon of coconut oil. But that goes a long way in the pan to sauté onions and garlic and your meats and your veggies and actually makes cooking and preparing a meal very, very nice.

The coconut oil also doubles as a body lotion to moisturize your skin because you can't use any makeup, any lotions, any oils, any shampoos. The point is we're trying to rid your body of all the chemicals that cause you to gain weight. So, a lot of people ask, "What the heck am I going to use?"

Now there are some organic soaps and organic toothpaste and shampoo you can use throughout the protocol and it's just a small sacrifice for a great and huge benefit.

Not only can you cook with it, but also you can actually put it on your skin and it works wonders for all things. I had a rash that I would break out with and when I did the HCG diet it killed off the rash.

The coconut oil, along with the diet protocol and the clean living, actually killed the rash off. It's really important to get the coconut oil. It will save you in the long run because people always complain about the food is dry, they can't cook with just lemon juice. That's an important thing to know.

HCG Body for Life Food Choices

Download Our HCG Body for Life Food Chart

http://tinyurl.com/hcgbflfoods

When following our Advanced HCG Body for Life protocol your food choices might appear slightly limited. After all, you will be ingesting around 550 calories with a maximum of 750 calories on days that you implement our strength training exercises. Exercising forces your body to release between 1,500 – 2,500 or more calories every day of compulsory excess fat stores. The other part of the equation (other than HCG itself) is the types of foods you eat to provide your body with the required 550 calories. These have been identified as the foods that will return you to your ideal weight set point.

The Importance of Food Quality…

Some say that it is critical that the foods you do eat must be pristine and organic. The reason for this argument is partly due to the chemical adulterants, preservatives and pesticides found in many commercially processed foods. Research has been shown that these chemicals are some of the main causes why our body's natural supply of HCG is depleted in the first place. Although most people will lose weight without eating organically; organic HCG Body for Life dieting appears to deliver better overall weight loss results than chemically process foods.

Getting Started On the HCG Body for Life Diet…

In the morning you'll be limited to unsweetened, **organic black coffee or solid tea** (one table spoon of milk is allowed however, or Lucerne Non-Fat Sugar Free creamer is an option). You have a number of options when it comes to tea:

Again, it is critical that the water used has been filtered and purified to remove any contaminants such as chlorine or fluoride; both are common in typical city water supplies.

Let's Do Lunch and Dinner…

When designing our program, like Dr. Simeons we identify pure proteins that aid in restoring balance to the body. These **lean**

meats, **beef, bison, veal,** should be of the organic free-range type whenever possible, Free-range, organic beef which are accessible at featured item in most whole Foods grocery stores and can be more costly than its conventionally counterpart. The other protein options are

- **White Fish**
- **Sea Bass**
- **Cod**
- **Crab Meat**
- **Flounder**
- **Haddock**
- **Halibut**
- **Lobster**
- **Red Snapper**
- **Shrimp**
- **Tilapia**
- **Lemon Sole**
- **Monk Fish**

- **Whiting**
- **Scallops,**
- **Lean Turkey**
- **Chicken Breast**

You need to avoid types of fish that are high in mercury like, deep-sea cold-water fish such as salmon tuna or Icelandic cod and salmon

Of course, you will need your servings of fruits and vegetables as well. Along with your beef serving, you can select any one of the following:

Remember not to add any kind of fat (such as butter or oil) other than your 1 tsp. of **organic coconut oils**. They can be either grilled, boiled, oven baked or steamed.

Fruit choices include…

You must not add sugar to the however Stevia is a great replacement.

- **Apples**
- **Strawberries**

- **Grapefruit**

It is also recommended, like your meat, poultry and fish, that your fruit and vegetables be organic as well whenever possible.

Vegetables

Choose from:

- **Spinach**
- **Chard**
- **Chicory**
- **Beet Greens**
- **Lettuce**
- **Tomatoes**
- **Celery**
- **Fennel**
- **Onions**
- **Radishes**
- **Cucumbers**
- **Asparagus**
- **Broccoli**

- **Zucchini**
- **Cabbage**
- **Chives**
- **Brussels Sprouts**
- **Mushrooms**

Do mix different types of vegetables in a serving. Some people find some combinations of vegetables bring larger daily releases than others while others find that some of this vegetable inhibits their weight loss. Asparagus, chives, zucchini and broccoli work well and can produce a diuretic effect, which could help to release excess fluids from your body.

Something to Remember…

It's undeniably critical to make sure that your diet is amply diverse from one day to the next. For example, if you eat Sea Bass and spinach for lunch; you'll want to have chicken and cucumbers for dinner, and then maybe, beef and tomatoes for lunch the following day.

Chicken and cucumbers for dinner, and then maybe, beef and tomatoes for lunch the following day.

Liquid or powder stevia

This is going to be your sweetener of choice and very few people have said that they don't like it. But stevia is your lifesaver because my wife Jayne has created some amazing deserts in Phase 3 that you would die for not using any sugars.

I'm talking about Key Lime pie, a strawberry, banana and raspberry tart with nuts as the crust. I could go on and on. It's amazing. But stevia is also what you can put on your strawberries and grapefruit, and on your apples with some cinnamon on it. And basically make your desserts after your meals in Phase 2 delicious and you can stay within the protocol without feeling that you are missing out on anything.

Green tea
Woolong tea
Yerba-Mate tea

Green teas not only help with your appetite, they help speed up your metabolism.

You're going to want to use these teas and mix them together if you like. You can drink them all day long to make sure your appetite stays under control. Depending on how much energy they're exerting some dieters may feel bouts of hunger and these teas help suppress their appetite.

Multivitamin

A multivitamin is optional. However it is recommended for those who may be anemic, or who have maintained previous diets low in vegetables. To be honest with you, I believe that all the green vegetables and protein you're eating gives all the nutrients you need. I've had people suggest that taking a multivitamin has been very beneficial to many dieters on the protocol.

I'm going to throw it out there because you know what -- you know, just because it doesn't apply to me, it may apply to other people. You may want to choose your best multivitamin you can find and to take it daily.

Acetyl L-Carnitine

Great supplement. This supplement helps take your fat and transform it into energy. It's going to actually take away some of the lethargy that people get sometimes on this diet.

Some people react differently to the diet. For me, my energy level was crazy; I was bouncing off the walls. On most days, I was on the treadmill in the morning and I was jogging at night because I just had too much energy.

Jayne on the other hand was dragging for the first five or seven days. The L-Carnitine is going to give you energy, help mobilize fat, and help you with your weight loss. It's going to help release that fat, turn it into energy.

And anything we can do to push the scale from 1 pound a day average to a pound and a half to 2 pounds can make a huge difference in your weight loss depending if you're doing a 26-day cycle or a 43-day cycle. You'll want to take L-Carnitine as a part of your daily regimen. It's excellent.

Vitamin B6 or vitamin B12

Take vitamin B6 or vitamin B12 either via shots or methyl-B12, which is used under the tongue. Some people have suggested that they've gotten better weight loss by mixing their HCG shot with a vitamin B12 shot.

Methyl Vitamin B same thing, but it goes under your tongue so it's like your sublingual vitamin B. That is another option. I personally like the B12 shots, and used them the last time I completed the protocol. It not only improves the weight loss but is also helped with Jayne's energy levels and helped her to feel great on the protocol during our last phase.

If you have an opportunity to implement the B12, then do so. I have gotten tons of feedback from our members who highly recommend it as well. I highly recommend adding B12 to you HCG diet regiment because it has clearly helped many dieters with their energy levels, weight loss, and overall feeling of wellbeing.

Unfiltered apple cider vinegar or Braggs

Braggs is a pure amino acid. It actually is kind of salty. It takes the place of salt. If you're sensitive to salt this will take the place of salt and also give you flavor on your vegetables.

And the apple cider vinegar is actually very, very good for your body. It helps with acid reflux. It also helps with your digestion. Some people after a week or two of having just apple cider vinegar on their vegetables find it difficult to endure throughout the entire protocol.

Having the Braggs as a backup to swap them out is a tremendous asset to you. You definitely need to have the apple cider vinegar or the Braggs liquid amines to put on your vegetables unless you like them plain and dry. I recommend that you sauté your vegetables with coconut oil, onions and garlic.

Mastering HCG Diet - Phase 3

This section is about phase 3, why it's important, and what you need to know about it in order for you to succeed at it.

If you want to listen to this information, you can listen to it by going to our channel on Blog Talk Radio and playing back those segments.

Audio link==→ Download audio: http://tinyurl.com/25w9vz9

Phase 3 is called the stabilization phase. I call it the muscle building phase because this is the phase where the transformation really took place and my body actually changed and I built up a lot of muscle in that phase. The reason why it's so important is because this is the phase in which you reset your hypothalamus gland which controls pretty much all the major things about you.

It controls your height, your weight, your eye color, and your waistline. I mean everything that determined our set point weight at birth. We were designed to be a certain height and a certain weight and we destroyed and basically manipulated our set point and pushed it out of whack by making poor eating choices and having a western diet.

This protocol is going to detox your body, reset your hypothalamus, and increase your metabolism to where it's normal for you. The goal is, through phase 3, is to reset your hypothalamus gland so you never gain the weight back.

Now, I say you'll never gain the weight back but that doesn't just come miraculously. You have to obviously have a lifestyle change. If you return to eating the way you ate before and doing the things you did before, your body is going to react the same as it did before. In other words, if you do the same thing, you will get the same results.

This is an opportunity for you to see what you are supposed to look like, feel how you are supposed to feel, and make a conscious choice and say, "I don't want to go back." That's why I call HCG Body for Life because you're getting a second chance to change your life. To change your body, the way you feel, and to live a longer life just by making the right choices.

What we're going to cover is what phase 3 is all about, why it's important, how to do it correctly, how to ease into the phase 3 and how to maximize it for muscle building.

Phase 3 is a stabilization phase. This is where you're going to stabilize your weight. And during the protocol, once you have left phase 2 and you've lost all the weight you can lose, and you've used up all your stored fat, you're going to go into phase 3. This is where you have a two-pound rule, which means you cannot lose two pounds or gain more than two pounds in the next 21 days of phase 3 because this is the period where you set your hypothalamus.

Now, if you allow your weight to go beyond two pounds, you're allowing the weight-set-point to set its own point, which is going to try to return back to previously calibrated weight. It doesn't matter if you lost 20 pounds or 200 pounds; you need to set your weight set point at this stage of the diet.

How do you do that? You may ask…you are going to go from your 550-750 calorie diet, and you're going to gradually take your body toward your natural BMR, which is your basal metabolic rate.

That is a rate in which your body burns your calories and produces energy for your level of activity. Everybody has their own number and I put a formula together that I found that makes it really easy for people to be able to calculate those numbers very quickly and know what your goal is as far as your BMR. What this means is the amount of calories you need to take in to gain weight, maintain your weight, or lose weight.

Everyone has heard of the phrase, calories in, and calories out. If you burn more calories than you take in, you'll lose weight. If you take in more calories than you burn, you'll gain weight.

And if you've taken the right amount of calories, you'll maintain your weight. That's the secret. It's not rocket science but it seems to elude all of us.

By implementing this formula and gradually, and I repeat, GRADUALLY taking yourself from your very low-calorie intake diet of 650 calories and gradually taking yourself up to where your maximum BMR is, you're going to be able to stabilize your weight.

Dr. Simeons put together a great protocol. He provided a lot of questions and answers but he did fail to explain to people how to correctly implement phase 3 because – They go from having 500 calories to apperception that there is no calorie limit... Believing they can eat anything they want as long as there is no sugars or starches in their diet.

Well, that could be a recipe for danger and disaster because some of my favorite foods are nuts. I love walnuts, peanuts -- peanut butter is one of my favorite foods.

Well, guess what, peanut butter is very high in calories and if I can sit there and just eat peanut butter all day long with all my other calories, I could easily consume 3,000 to 4,000 calories. What would happen if I eat 3,000 or 4,000 calories too soon in phase 3, I would start storing fat again in the same places where it just left. Therefore, it's very important that you take it very slowly.

How do you do this? It's very simple. If you're going from a 650-calorie diet, you're going to gradually increase your calories in increments of 500 or 600 depending on your goal weight and your maximum BMR, to reach your final calorie intake.

For example, if you're a woman and your end weight on the last day that you weighed yourself in phase 2 is 145 pounds, you would multiply that by 11, which come out to be about 1,595 pounds. You would round that off to 1,600 calories, okay?

That means that your maximum daily caloric intake for your body at this new weight is 1,600. Anything over that will cause you to gain weight anything under that you'll continue to lose weight but if you maintain a range of 1,600 or 1,500 calories a day, you'll maintain the weight that you have.

You've been very conscious about 650 calories for the last 26 days or 43 days depending on which protocol you did so you've already created this habit. Now it's about just continuing the habit and staying within the guidelines.

Phase 3 states that you can now introduce dairy, cheese, milk, eggs back into the diet, but you can't have any sugar, any starch. Keep in mind, there are spreads, pastas and potatoes that are considered starchy vegetables or food, so keep this in mind.

Breakfast cereals, whole grain breads, and all the general stuff that you think are still good for you cannot be consumed. Everything else is on the table. All the vegetables that you want (that you weren't able to eat before) like mushrooms and some of the foods you weren't able to eat before like bananas, can now be eaten but you still need to control how many calories you're taking in.

You do that by just being conscious and figuring out how many calories you're taking in. If you do that, you won't struggle so much in this maintenance phase or go two pounds up or two pounds down.

If you go over two pounds in the 21 days of phase 3, you have to do what's called the "steak day or apple day." The steak day looks like this.... you have to fast throughout the entire day and then eat a steak along with either a raw tomato or an apple. The apple day you will eat 6 apples (only apples) throughout the day.

This will take your weight set point back to where you were when you finished the diet. It works very magically and it works every single time but the point is it's not very pleasant if you have to do it every other day.

The point is paying attention and gradually increasing your calories. As an example, there was a young lady that finished her protocol at 145 pounds. She knew her calories should now be 1,595 calories. She would go from 500 calories to 750 the first week and stayed within that range for the very first week, to allow her body to gradually get used to the increased calories.

From week 2 and week 3 she went from 750 to 1,100 and steadily increasing more food. At this stage she was also bringing in more fats and proteins into her diet. The last week she raised her calories from 1,100 to 1,595 or 1,600 calories. Now her body had gradually gotten used to the increase in calories.

The same thing applies with men. The formula for men is your last weigh-in weight, multiplied by 12, and that gives you your maximum metabolic rate.

If you weighed 190 at the end of your protocol, you'd multiply that x12 and you'd have calories of 2,290 calories and that is your maximum daily intake of calories.

No sugars, no starches are allowed but you would increase your calories from 500 to 1,100 and from 1,100 to 1,600, from 1,600 to 2,200. You would basically increase by 600 calories. You can easily reach your calorie requirement and enjoy a lot of different things.

What is really important about this phase is that once you stabilize your hypothalamus and then reset your weight set point and your metabolism, you're going to be able to go into phase 4. You'll be able to actually reintroduce different combinations of foods, like carbohydrates, fats, and sugars, back into your life.

I believe this entire process is going to be a spiritual process. You're going to find out things about yourself you really didn't know. It's going to expose your triggers. You're going to expose the things that make you eat when you're not hungry.

As you take all this information, all this knowledge and you actually implement it and learn it, learn about yourself then you're going to realize that you're going to have to ask yourself the following question. "Look, I've done such a great job. I worked so hard to get this new body. I feel great. Do I want to start putting this poison back into my system?"-

"Do I want to start eating candy bars and refined sugar? Do I want to start eating processed foods?" You know, I think that if you can't read the label or the label has three or four words on it that you can't pronounce, don't eat it.

You have to eat fresh food, fresh fruit, fresh vegetables, lean proteins, and on occasion fatty desserts. Indulge yourself occasional you're learning how to implement new habits in your life to maintain your weight. There is no magic cure here to keep the weight off for the rest of your life unless you're equally committed to maintaining some of these lessons that you have learned throughout the process.

To maintain your weight, and stay within the two-pound rule it is important to adhere to, this phase of the protocol just as diligently as you implemented phase 2. Not doing so, could be another recipe for disaster and inevitable weight gains.

Now I want to talk about the point of actually using this phase to burn more fat and build muscle. A lot of people ask me, "I saw your before, middle, and after photos and seems like you got really muscular at the end of this phase. What did you do differently?"

People have asked me point blank... "I see other people lost weight, and they look great but it doesn't seem like they gained any muscle". Well, my putting on more muscle was done intentionally. This was intentional because once I got the green light in phase 3 to increase my protein and vegetables, and calorie intake, and used these extra foods to increase my muscle mass in phase 3. With some hard work, and our MAX-26 HIIT (High Intensity Interval Training) workouts, these HIIT circuit-training exercises helped Jayne and I both to really pack on the muscle quickly.

Most people fail to take advantage of this opportunity to make sure that they have utilized all of their stored fat. If you've actually taken this protocol to the limit where your body signals you that you have exhausted all of your abnormal fat stores, then you are in a perfect position to build more muscle in phase 3. However, if you've chosen to just take the protocol to the point where you simply feel good about yourself, and are comfortable with your image in the mirror then these are two very different stages.

The diet is designed to use up all your stored fat. How you know you've actually completed the protocol successfully is because while you're on HCG, and eating your 550 to 750 calories, you will no longer be able to maintain this low calorie diet. You will feel like you're starving.

HCG has this magical way of releasing fat into your bloodstream at 2,000-3,000 and sometimes up to 7,000 calories a day that your body uses for energy.

What happens if your fat bank is gone? What happens if you've exhausted it? There's nowhere for it to pull from so the only thing left is going to be muscle. But before it goes after your muscles it's going to warn you. It's going to say, "You're hungry. You're starving."

There's a huge difference between psychological hunger and true physical hunger. The average person cannot sustain a 650-calorie diet without some sort of assistance either through some sort of appetite suppressant (and I don't think it really works) but HCG seems to work miraculously in that category. So once it stops working for you then you have completed the protocol successfully. That means you've used up all the stored fat.

If you follow the protocol and you increase your protein intake to around a gram per pound of body weight per day of protein (man or a woman), because that's what's sufficient for you in order to build muscle, you actually complete the transformation and turn your body into a fat burning machine that looks strong, healthy and muscular.

You can transform your body to whatever physique you want by utilizing the stages of this protocol.

You can recreate the physique you want and it doesn't matter how old you are. I'm 48 years old. I'm going to be 49 years old in a few weeks and I'm in as good a shape as I was in my 20s.

Now, does that tell you your body has a memory? My body remembered what I was supposed to be and took me back there. That means everyone's has the same genetics within him or her. What I always like to say..."Everybody has an HCG body within them"

I really want you to know that transformation is absolutely possible with our HCG Body for Life protocol and all you have to do is follow it. Don't reinvent the wheel and don't try to outsmart it because you're going to only outsmart yourself. It is simple as reading the protocol, getting what you need, getting the tools you need to prepare for it, and then following it to the letter and letting it do what it's got to do and just bless the process.

I guarantee you that you'll build the body and a level of health that you have never seen.

One thing also that's miraculous about this is that I was a smoker for years. I smoked cigars for years. I was a heavy drinker. I mean I had all the bad habits you can imagine in my lifetime. One thing about the HCG Body for Life protocol is that it just doesn't kill off your food cravings. It also can kill off cravings for alcohol and tobacco. So if you're someone who is just the personification of non-health, you can take this opportunity to not only get rid of the drinking habit or at least minimize your drinking habit, absolutely get rid of the smoking habit and get rid of the crazy food cravings you have and do it all at one time, completely detoxify your body and get a brand new life.

I don't know what it is about this substance but it has the ability to subdue the cravings. I just want to invite you to the possibility that whatever your bad habits are, whatever the things you want to change about yourself that has to do with your physical health and physical wellbeing, then take advantage of this protocol.

The two-pound rule

Some people have the tendency to think, "It's only two pounds. I was letting go of three pounds or four pounds."

Your steak or apple day has got to be done on your very first morning that you noticed you've hit over two pounds. If you do not, it's too late. Now you've allowed your weight set point to creep to another level instead of where it's supposed to be. Then it will be on maximum level but it's another level and the steak or apple day is not as effective.

This is not a protocol that is designed for you to turn into a yo-yo diet. It works. I don't fear gaining weight because I know I can lose it.

But the point is you want to work on changing your thought process about your goal and just maintaining your health versus having that feeling where, "Oh, man, I was there and I blew it and I got to do it all over again."

Starting over is not easy. You know what I'm talking about. Just be very careful and know that you can actually gain weight. If you look in the mirror and look the same for a very long period of time, then all of a sudden it changes, then the reason is that your body is starting to store fat again in all those places and it's coming in evenly and so you don't realize the gradual increase in size.

Remember that it's very important that you follow this protocol all the way through. Follow phase 1. Do the gorging. Follow phase 2; the very low-calorie diet to the letter. Follow phase 3 and use these tips about gradually increasing your calories. This will limit your frustration of having to do a steak or apple day every other day of just blowing it out and letting your hypothalamus reset at the wrong place.

Mastering HCG Diet - Phase 4

Audio link==→ Download audio: http://tinyurl.com/2g5n3m3

Now we're going to be covering Phase 4 or what is called learning to eat to live instead of living to eat. Creating new eating habits for life; it's ironic that this is the question that people ask me the most before they start the protocol "Okay, great. I lose weight but how do I keep it off?"

Some of the points we're going to be covering are, "how do we introduce starches and sugars back into our diet and not gain weight?" which are basically your carbohydrates, back into your diet.

We're also going to cover eating to live instead of living to eat, which is something that I think most of us do. This section will also deal with portion control, which is really the key to maintaining your weight loss and also maintaining some of the habits that you're going to learn (or you've already learned depending on what phase you're in with the protocol).

When we talk about sugars and starches, we're really talking about carbohydrates, and this is the danger zone for a lot of people because if we're introducing these carbs or these sugars or starches too quickly, it can actually cause weight again.

The goal is that you don't want to gain more than two pounds from your newly reset hypothalamus weight – body weight. And obviously, if you put the wrong foods or the wrong combination of foods in your body too quickly, you're going to see some weight gains.

What are carbohydrates?

There are simple carbohydrates and long-acting carbohydrates, but carbs can be basically beans, breads, pastas, popcorns, potatoes, oatmeal, cookies, and soft drinks; cherry pie, your fruit juices, even milk and yogurts, also fall in this category as well as other sweets.

By themselves, they're not really bad things. They're actually very essential to our body. They control our blood sugar. Almost all carbs break down into sugars, and then some of those sugars can either spike your blood sugar or stabilize your blood sugar depending on which carbs we use.

We have to have carbs in our diet in order to balance out diet. The problem is that some of us are more sensitive to some carbs and less sensitive to others. I'm sensitive to starchy carbs and if I eat too many of them in the wrong combinations, I will find that body will tend to gain weight.

The basic building blocks of carbohydrates are sugars and they have to be broken down into sugars so our body can assimilate them. We also need these carbs for our daily energy, also for muscle growth when we're exercising therefore; we have to put carbs as well as proteins into our body to maintain a sensible diet.

In Phase 3 when we talked about gradually increasing your calorie intake from 650 calories to 800 to 1500, to whatever your natural daily calorie intake should be.

Carbs are going to be very much the same way. As we talked about it in Phase 3, it's a three-week stabilization phase, 21 days.

Now, we're going to continue with that week with week 4, 5 and 6 and this will complete stabilizing your weight and getting used to going back into your normal eating habits.

I'm sure you've heard that it takes 21 days to either break a habit or create a new one. What have you been doing for, the last 26- to 43-days in phase 2?

You've been measuring your portions.

You've been eating fruits and vegetables, and if you've been combining your vegetables like we do here, then you're probably having six servings of vegetables, six to nine servings of vegetables a day.

You're having your lean proteins. You're having your simple carbs, which is your fruits, your fresh fruits, your apple, your strawberries, and your grapefruits. And you basically have been having a very balanced diet, but you've also been having very controlled portions.

We do our portions a little bit differently when we do the HCG Body for Life diet. They are very full and they're actually very filling, but we're not stuffed at the end of the process. The goal is to maintain this same level of portion control as you move into your normal eating pattern, as you move into Phase 3 and then

Phase 4.

Something that a lot of people don't realize is that, sometimes we don't pay attention to our portions. The success for keeping the weight off for the rest of your life is really just being present.

You have to measure your food. You have to prepare your food. You have to take your time to figure out exactly what you're going to eat, how much you're going to eat, and when is the next time you're going to eat. And guess what? You're present.

You're paying attention to what you're putting into your body and how it's going into your body and how much is going into your body. What happens when we're off of a diet, when we're off of some sort of protocol, we usually are reaching and grabbing for whatever impulse that we have, not paying attention or counting the calories that we intake. What happens usually is that we take in more calories than our body can process in any one day. And where is it going to go? It's going to be stored as fat.

Keep this in mind as we move into week 4. This is the very first week out of your maintenance phase and if you've successfully completed your maintenance phase, you can get on the scale and your weight should be stable. You won't see your body weight dramatically jumping in either direction. Rather, you should see moderate changes in weight on a daily bases staying within two pounds. This will be a clear indication to you that you have successfully reset you metabolism.

Now it's time to start to re-introduce sugars or starches. For example, say that you have missed bread what you want to do is eat your bread but you're going to have it in one meal, you're going to have your bread and that's one day.

The next day, you're going to introduce a different starch or sugar and that would be one of your meals but only have it once.

This keeps you conscious and <u>present</u> again, but also your body is getting used to slowly processing these sugars, carbs and starches back into your system.

It also lets you know which sugars or starches your body is sensitive to, because as you move forward you're going to continue to weigh yourself on a daily basis. I do it every day. It's just a part of my routine. I get up in the morning. I go to the bathroom. I get on the scale to check my weight, and that lets me know how the day before went.

By doing this, you'll notice that if you eat a baked potato or a sugary cereal, you'll know if your body reacts to it. You can actually write it down and keep a log of the foods that your body reacts adversely or positively to.

I was sensitive to baked potatoes so I'm going to limit the amount of baked potatoes I have throughout my week or throughout my month, but at least you don't have to eliminate it completely, now you have an idea of how your body is reacting these foods.

For the entire week of that fourth week, you're going to introduce one new starch or sugar into your diet a day, very simple. Now, you get to enjoy whatever it is you've been missing and thought you'll never have again, but instead of having it all the time, you're having it once throughout the day.

As you move into week 5, you're going to have two carbs together, but you're not going to eat them at the same meal. Now, you get to enjoy two different carbs, either your starch or your sugary carb, but now you're going to have them at different times, so not the same meal, but now you get to have two in a day.

And you do that same thing for the next week, introducing different starches and different sugars into your diet and watching how your body reacts to it, okay? So you do that for the entire next week. What happens when you do things like that over a 7-day period, not only are you paying attention to what's your body is doing, not only are you present, but you're also realizing what foods your body is sensitive to, which ones work for you and which ones don't.

Then as you move into week 6, you're going to now combine your carbs in the same meal. Now, you can actually have oatmeal and your toast. You got two basic starchy carbs in the same meal. You've got to pay attention to your body. You're also introducing your body slowly to something new and you're going to see how it reacts.

Once you've completed three weeks of doing this, you pretty much would have had every sugary carb or starchy carb that you normally would eat, eliminating whatever you think is just your Achilles' heel.

If there are certain foods, then say to yourself, "Look, you know what? Once in a blue moon, I'm going to have this type of food because it's just not good for me."

What happens is a change in the way you look at food, and eating in general. After you've been eating clean, your body has been detoxed from sugars and certain cravings, and it's your choice if you want to awaken the beast from within or you're going to let the sleeping dog lie.

If you know that you had a weakness, then guess what? Be intelligent to say, "Look, I'm just going to bypass that and choose..." You know, choose another poison if you will. I always say choose your poisons.

You can choose one that makes you sick or choose one that's deadly. And so I'll choose the ones that will make me sick versus deadly, and that just gives you a briefing if you know who you are, and you know how you are when it comes to certain foods.

But after you've now gone through the process of reintroducing these foods back into your system, you're going to make choices of some foods you're going to skip for life or at least skip for quite some time. You want to also avoid overeating.

Your body has its own natural maximum calorie intake for maintaining your weight. If you exceed that on a regular basis, you will gain weight. If you reduce your calories on a regular basis, you will lose weight, and this is the way for you to actually control where you want to be as far as your weight is concerned.

That same premise has to be in place when you start introducing other foods that you've not had for quite some time. You want to still make sure you're staying within your daily calorie intake.

If you splurge on a certain sugary food, as long as you're staying within your maximum calorie intake for that particular day and you're conscious if that's the situation you made, then the very next day, you can correct that by eating healthier, you're still going to maintain your weight.

It's about being conscious and paying attention. I'm not saying you have to weigh every single thing you eat and count every single calorie. It's almost impossible really to count calories accurately, but the point is that most of us gain weight and our weight gets out of control, because we live unconsciously.

We open cabinets and pick up foods and open packages and eat them without even paying attention. If you're going to have some chips, reach and take a handful of chips, put it on a napkin, close the bag up, walk away, sit down, eat those chips.

If you have the bag in front of you, you're going to unconsciously just eat the entire bag. If you're going to have a slice of cake, then get a slice of cake and eat the cake seated someplace else. Just savor that moment that you enjoyed it and ignore the impulse to go back and have another piece because you really don't need it.

Overeating issues

Let's talk about the overeating issues because it happens. Try to avoid putting both high fat and high-carb meals together.

The food industry has put certain foods together that actually are poor combinations that cause us to get fat. I mean you could have chips and salsa, which is a starchy chip or a starchy carb and have some salsa, but when you take the chip salsa and you add guacamole,(even though avocados are good for you), it's considered a high fat.

Even if it was a good fat, it's still a high-fat food. You put that combination together and all of a sudden that combination becomes highly caloric and highly fattening.

Paying attention to how you're putting your foods together can make a huge difference between maintaining your weight and gaining your weight back. It's not like it's difficult. It's just about trying to remember how conscious you were about losing the weight, how conscious you were about maintaining your weight and just don't throw it all away when you get to the point where now, you have a free for all to eat whatever you can.

One habit I think you should keep for life is weighing yourself every day. It gives you an indication if you had too much sodium the day before or too much of anything, because anything in excess is going to cause a problem.

When you get away with it or you get used to doing it, it becomes a new habit. And you want to remove the bad habits and embrace the new ones that are on a path of healthy living.

When you're on the scale, it actually reminds you, "Whoa! Yesterday was a little much with the margaritas and the chips and the salsa. Consequently today, I'm going to have a low-carb, low-fat diet day and guess what? I'll balance out tomorrow." And that's really the way to do it.

It also counts when you travel. Take out an extra pair of shoes and put it in your scale. Because when you're on vacation, this can be the kiss of death. Every time that Jayne and I gained weight off of the protocol, we were not living at home. When we're away, it is difficult trying to eat at buffets because you have it all-inclusive.

You have the drinks. You have the food, but you can still limit the portions you have even at a buffet. You can go back as much as you want and all the foods are usually bad combinations. You need to be very careful which combinations you choose.

But when you don't have a scale, all of a sudden you come back and you're 10 pounds heavier than you were when you left. Those 10 pounds may not show up immediately in your clothes or in the mirror, but it's the part that just sneaks up on you.

All of a sudden 10 pounds becomes 15 pounds, and you realize it when your pants get too tight or your skirt gets too tight. Thus in order to avoid that, have the scale with you. Everything is a conscious choice. If you want to drink all the margaritas you want one day and eat all the fattening food you want that day, celebrate. Have a great time. The next day, you can just be conscious and cut it back a bit and maintain your weight set point.

It's the same thing with restaurant eating. Many times you go to a restaurant and you don't realize that the portions you're getting are designed for two. There's something that Jayne and I do almost every time that we dine out. We find a meal that we both like, foods we both enjoy, and we split the meal, we usually order a big salad, and we split the salad and we end up having the right portion for us. We walk away from the table feeling completely satisfied, not overstuffed, and guess what, we don't take a doggy bag. There's nothing to consume at 12:00 at night when you get home. And that's a very easy way to make sure that you still maintain the similar portions you would when you're eating at home versus when you're out.

People don't realize that it takes about 30 minutes for your body to process or feel the feeling of hunger, and for cravings for food to subside. What happens is that most of us don't take 30 minutes to eat a meal.

We usually wolf it down as it comes and then we're pretty much done within 10 to 15 minutes. By the time you've actually finished the meal, you've already overstuffed. How many times do you walk away from the table going "Oh, man, I ate too much."

You feel uncomfortable and you just want to unbutton your pants. You want to lay down someplace. If you don't think it feels good, it doesn't feel good for a reason because of the fact that you have overloaded your body.

In most cases, you probably have overloaded your calorie intake for the day as well. Therefore make a mental note of this. I'm just giving you a bunch of things you could think about while you're living your life.

If you think of food as sustenance and as necessary fuel for your body in order for you to function it is much easier for you to maintain your weight.

The bottom line is eating to a point where you're full. Feel the feeling of being full and then stop. It's always better to take a smaller portion and go back and get another one, if you really need it.

Filling your plate up with all the stuff you think you're going to have and then trying to polish it off, that's where you're going to find some problems. We are told this as kids "Don't leave the table till you're done". I don't think our parents really realize that by forcing us to eat beyond what we were capable of, and beyond that capacity of being full, that they actually were preparing us to overeat for the rest of our lives.

Portion control is still the key. It doesn't matter if you're at a friend's barbecue or if you're at a restaurant or you're at home. If you can't measure it, then use the palm of your hand as the right portion of any given meal.

If you treat every dish like a sampler and you have just a little of everything, you get all the flavors of all the foods you want but you've maintained the portions. You're not going to have any problems keeping your new weight set point and controlling your weight. I just want you to keep this in mind.

Know your limitations.

A balanced nutritious diet includes the proteins, the carbs, the fats and the sugars. The bottom line is that skipping any one thing from your diet completely is going to leave you unbalanced.

We need to have all those types of foods except for the processed foods and the foods that have names and ingredients can't pronounce. I learned not too long ago, actually, a little over two years ago, that if you pick up a package, and you read the label, and you feel that you need a degree in chemistry to know what's in it… Don't buy it! This made a lot of sense me.

If you're picking up a can or a bag and you can't read the words that sound like a chemical, it's a pretty good indication that it's not in your best interest to consume it.

And guess what? The stuff that's not in your best interest to consume tastes the best. There's no mistake in that, there's a reason for it. We can either be fooled by the food industry and eat the junk or we can be conscious and eat real food. If you eat real food, that means real fruits, real vegetables, what you've been basically doing with the HCG body for life diet.

"Choose to be in Close Proximity to People who are Empowering ... Who See the Greatness in You!" ~Wayne Dyer

Your portion limitations can now be increased to where it's normal for your normal calorie intake. When you're off the diet, you're not going to have any problem maintaining your weight. It is not rocket science.

You're just being present and paying attention to the most important part of you, which is basically staying healthy. I think anyone who goes through this protocol and has the discipline to complete it and goes through the phases will look amazing and feel amazing.

Nothing feels more empowering than being in control and beating the demons that have been beating you for your entire life. The best way to do this is just to take heed and follow the principals of the protocol. Take them in, practice them and make them a part of your life, and you're going to be perfectly fine.

I'm just going to recap so you can get the big trigger points:

- Add your starches and sugars gradually.
- put your combinations together one week at a time, not

one day at a time.
- eat to live and not live to eat.

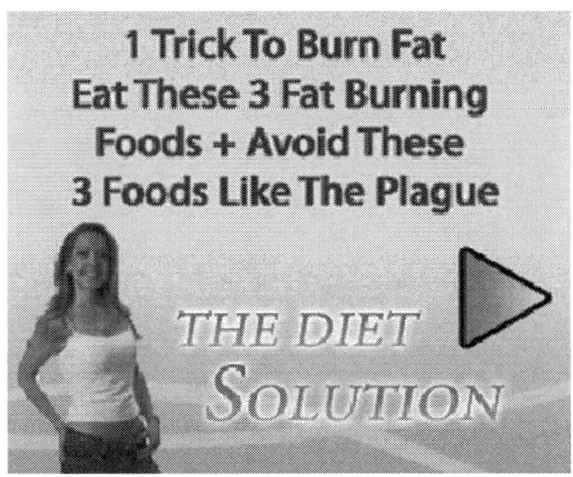

Just be conscious and present. Portion control is the key to success and maintaining any balanced weight and body shape. You need to maintain the habits that you've learned throughout the weeks that you've been on the protocol and you'll live and have a HCG Body for Life.

The best phase 4-maintenance plan I have found, and have personally used to maintain my lean body is The Diet Solution Plan. This is a simple easy to follow and implement for everyday life. I highly recommend that you invest in this program to help you maintain your new healthy HCG Body. Here a link to review this program. **http://tinyurl.com/dietsolution22**

Food & Supplement Choices

Introduction

This is one of the most important chapters in the entire book, because it takes you far beyond what most people do (or are prepared to do) on a regular basis.

Changing your nutritional intake is a conscious decision and requires a conscious effort to maintain. It is much easier to resort back to easy snacks and microwave dinners, but this is something that you must decide for yourself to avoid doing.

A change in your eating habits is essential and this could translate into major weight loss, lower body fat, better productivity, higher energy levels, and your achieving the ultimate success in life (eating quality foods goes far beyond just body image).

Foods that feed the fat burning aspect of the body will let you lose maximum body fat in the least amount of time. If you can supply such a stream of nutrients then your life will improve exponentially (in emotional, intellectual and physical ways).

"We would not have to forgive people if we didn't judge them in the first place."
—Barry Neil Kaufman

Foods You Can Eat

Fruit

Fruit is a natural food and has been eaten for thousands of years. It simply needs to be picked and eaten raw.

Fruits contain lots of vital vitamins. Vitamin C is a powerful vitamin that the body needs to function.

Oranges and avocados also allow for better brain function and cell formation. This is known to minimize the risk of strokes.

Vegetables

Vegetables are the best source of antioxidants that the body needs. Antioxidants are known to prevent aging. The body actually contains very low amounts of antioxidants, so it needs to get as much as it can from food sources.

Antioxidants actually protect cells from damage from free radicals, which can be abundant in the brain (because it is so active). You can also find a lot of linoleic acid in leafy green veggies and olive oil.

Best Antioxidant Foods:

- Spinach
- Kale
- Strawberries
- Plums
- Grapefruit
- Tomato
- Orange
- Blueberries
- Cranberry

Foods to Avoid

Sugars and Starches

Carbohydrates are the danger zones. If you eat too many, too fast, you may gain a lot of weight. Hence to avoid that, this is what we have learned.

What Are Carbohydrates?

Carbohydrates are found in a wide array of foods such as bread, beans, milk, popcorn, potatoes, cookies, spaghetti, soft drinks, corn, and cherry pie.

They also come in a variety of forms. The most common and abundant forms are sugars, fibers, and starches.

The basic building block of every carbohydrate is a sugar molecule, a simple union of carbon, hydrogen, and oxygen. Starches and fibers are essentially chains of sugar molecules. Some contain hundreds of sugars. Some chains are straight, others branch wildly.

Carbohydrates were once grouped into two main categories.

Simple carbohydrates included sugars such as fruit sugar (fructose), corn or grape sugar (dextrose or glucose), and table sugar (sucrose).

Complex carbohydrates included everything made of three or more linked sugars. Complex carbohydrates were thought to be the healthiest to eat, while simple carbohydrates weren't so great. It turns out that the picture is more complicated than that.

The digestive system handles all carbohydrates in much the same way—it breaks them down (or tries to break them down) into single sugar molecules, since only these are small enough to cross into the bloodstream. It also converts most digestible carbohydrates into glucose (also known as blood sugar), because cells are designed to use this as a universal energy source.

Wanting security in a world where everything is inherently impermanent is a contradiction. There is wisdom in surrender to insecurity

How Much Food Is Allowed?

Measuring portions when eating regular meals is a habit you will have to develop during the HCG body for life diet, and it is a good one to keep. You do not need to be fanatical about measuring, but this will help you gauge how much food you are actually eating.

You will become accustomed to looking at food and know the portion size, and this will help you when you eat at restaurants. In most restaurants the portions are so large, that we do not realize we are usually eating two meals at one sitting.

Eating until the hunger sensation is gone, not until the "stuffed" sensation occurs is a problem many people have. It takes about 30 minutes for the satiety sensation (the sensation of being full) to set in after you have eaten a meal.

If you eat till you feel completely full, you have overstuffed yourself. Eat normal size portions and watch your caloric intake, and you will be able to be full without feeling like a stuffed pig.

"Eating to live, not living to eat." – This is the best advice I can give you. If you can begin to look at food as necessary fuel for your body instead of a treat, it will help you make the right choices. You will choose nutrient rich foods that will nourish your body over foods that are only made to satisfy the taste buds.

Supplements

Nutritional supplements are very important as part of the overall HCG body for life diet, as they give you many of the substances that your body needs. There are many things that will be listed, which you need to get from an external source (as your body cannot produce them).

There are also some symptoms that can be overcome by using nutritional supplements.

If you have symptoms such as fatigue, the inability to lose weight after extensive efforts, allergies, frequent influenza, arthritis, anxiety, depression, reduced memory, difficulties in concentrating and insomnia, you may be suffering from Adrenal Fatigue.

Other key signs and symptoms of Adrenal Fatigue may include salt cravings, elevated blood sugar under stress, increased PMS, increased pre-menopausal, or menopausal symptoms under stress, mild depression, lack of energy, decreased ability to handle stress, muscle weakness, absent mindedness, decreased sex drive, mild constipation alternating with diarrhea, as well as many others.

The onset of adrenal fatigue often occurs because of financial pressures, un-employment, infections, emotional stress, smoking, drugs, poor eating habits, sugar and white flour products, and several other stressors.

After experiencing many of these events over a long period of time, the adrenal glands become fatigued which may slow down metabolism leading to weight gain.

Nutritional supplements may offer benefits to participants experiencing Adrenal Fatigue symptoms. The following vitamins and minerals are recommended in addition to the Adrenal Tea Complex for dieters that may be suffering from Adrenal Fatigue: Vitamin C, Vitamin E w/mixed tocopherol, Vitamin B complex, Vitamin B-5 (Pantothenic acid), Niacin B-6, Magnesium citrate and Liquid trace minerals: *(zinc, manganese, selenium, chromium, molybdenum, copper, iodine)*All of the above nutrients are included in our recommended Pharmaceutical Multi-Vitamin/Mineral Supplement listed on the next pages.*

Recommended Supplements

We are now going to explore the most important supplements that you should include as part of your diet.

Laminine

WHAT IS Laminine™?

When we started down the path of looking to provide its customers a solid, proven nutritional supplement to aid the brain in regulating the body and build a stronger body, we searched for an amino acid and oligo peptide combination, which had all the required nourishment for the task at hand.

We found numerous studies for the cause and effect of individual amino acids, peptides and hormones, not to mention an equal number of products touting high dosages of one over another as beneficial for consumption. What was not clear was how many companies had developed and proven the right "combination" of amino acids, peptides, and growth factors required? It didn't surprise us to find there were none. So we embarked on our own research project. We looked for a balanced amino acid/peptide blend in nature, which could meet our needs with minimal additions.

Benefits may include:

- * Improve Energy
- * Burn Fat & Curbs Appetite
- * Elevate Serotonin Levels
- * Increase Clarity and Alertness
- * Increase Libido
- * Quicker Muscle Recovery
- * Increased Muscle Tone
- * Increased Muscle Strength

* Improve Stamina

* Aid in Brain Function

* Mood Enhancement

* Reduce Signs of Aging

* Reduce Stress

* Stimulate Natural DHEA

* Decrease Pain

* Build Collagen for Healthier Skin

* Stimulate Testosterone

Acetyl-L-Carnitine

http://tinyurl.com/L-Carnatine

What if there was one nutrient, which could help you lose weight, increase energy, lower cholesterol, and promote heart health? L-Carnitine does all that and more. L-Carnitine offers all these benefits by promoting fat burning. L-Carnitine is the only nutrient that can transport fat to the part of the cell that burns it off: the mitochondria. If you can't get fat into the mitochondria, you can't burn it. Without L-Carnitine, no fat burning can occur. Optimal L-Carnitine levels, on the other hand, allow our body to burn fat at an optimal rate.

L-Carnitine is sometimes called an amino acid, but it is not. It is similar in structure to B vitamins, especially choline. However, L-Carnitine is not a true vitamin because the body makes it in small amounts. L-Carnitine is also found in animal products, especially red meat. Unless you are eating pounds of red meat a day, however, you are probably not getting enough

L-Carnitine.

Signs of inadequate L-Carnitine intake include:
Fatigue

Progressive Weight Gain

High Cholesterol and Triglycerides

Weak Heart Function

Lack of Mental Focus

Poor Immune Function

Benefits of L-Carnitine:

Increases fat burning

Increases energy levels

Lowers cholesterol & triglycerides

Promotes health

Gives you more energy to exercise &

increases endurance & performance

Reduces food cravings

Promotes healthy circulation

Promoted liver health

Multi-Vitamin/Mineral Supplement

Vitamins and Minerals are an essential part of any weight loss program. They help maintain and support adequate nutrients to the tissues, cells and vital organs in the body. They also help in maintaining energy levels especially on a low calorie diet regiment.

http://tinyurl.com/MultiPlusMineralSup2

Contains: Vitamins A, B1, B2, B3, B5, B6, B12, C, D3, E, K1, Biotin, Calcium, Manganese, Iodine, Zinc, Selenium, Copper, Magnesium, Quercetin, Chromium, Folic Acid, Alpha Lipoic Acid, CoQ10, Green Tea Extract, Grape Seed Extract, Red Wine Extract, Resveratrol, Lutein, Black Pepper. * Do not use if allergic to Soy * *Recommended for a lifetime use*

"There is no passion to be found playing small - in settling for a life that is less than the one you are capable of living."
Nelson Mandela

Deep Acting Colon Cleanse

This is a highly potent, deep acting intestinal cleanse that contains a proprietary blend of herbs, vitamins, minerals, and amino acids to support easy intestinal elimination gently detoxifying the digestive tract, relieves bloating, slims the waistline and assists in weight loss with immediate results.

http://tinyurl.com/10DayColonCleanse

This product not only helps break up and remove impacted waste, but it prevents future buildup from occurring.

A deep acting proprietary herbal blend of calcium (from calcium carbonate)70 mg 7%, cascara segrada, fennel seed, ginger root, Irish moss, slippery elm bark, cayenne (capsicum), lactobacillus acidophilus cultures, barberry, bark root, soy, chlorella, licorice root, marshmallow root, raspberry powder root leaf and anise seed oil. (Recommended to be taken for 10 days on the first week of HCG therapy.)

Fat Burner/Thermogenic Modulator

http://tinyurl.com/Lipo10Thermagenic

Thermogenic agents may also promote **Fat Oxidization**. Fat oxidation means maintaining your lean muscle mass while you lose the pounds and inches. This is the key to maintaining a faster metabolism for long-term results.

Many of our coaching students (even after they reach their weight-loss goals) continue to take these natural pharmaceutical grade supplements. This will also help to maintain your results long term.

Adrenal Health Formula

http://tinyurl.com/AdrenalHealth
#

Some herbal remedies that have been noted as possible therapies include: Licorice, Ashwagandha, Astragalus Membranaceus, Siberian and Korean Ginseng.

We encourage our coaching students to order the Pharmaceutical Grade Adrenal Complex and Multi-Vitamin/Mineral Supplement to enhance weight loss and decrease adrenal fatigue and are highly recommended for any weight loss program.

This is also used to stimulate the immune system and the bodies' own ability to resist and combat most known diseases.

Pro-Biotic Formula

http://tinyurl.com/ProBiotic90

A daily maintenance Probiotic formula that promotes healthy digestive function is recommended. The supplement should contain multiple strains of micro flora, including bifidus bacteria, Lactobacilli, and Lactococcus cultures to support intestinal and immune health. These products should contain the following:

- At least 5 billion organisms per caplet
- Multiple strains of Bifidus bacteria, Lactobacilli, and Lactococcus cultures
- A guaranteed delivery of active cultures
- Dairy-free, gluten-free
- Shelf life-stable with no refrigeration necessary

Candida Colon Cleanse

http://tinyurl.com/CandidaCleanse

Candida Albicans is common yeast normally found in the digestive tract. This yeast can proliferate, upsetting the balance in the gastro-intestinal track, giving rise to problems such as rectal itching, diarrhea, constipation, bloating, skin problems, and many other issues.

The goal of the Candida Cleanse is to decrease the amount of yeast to a normal and manageable level. This product is formulated with all natural herbal and mineral ingredients used to support overgrowth of Candida yeast.

Ancient Tea

I don't have to tell you that it seems like everywhere you look there are people making outrageous claims about some new synthetic miracle pill that can help you fight the battle of the bulge.

You know we both despise that kind of junk.

And you probably also agree it sure is nice when you discover that something that is backed by dozens and dozens of lab studies and solid research that actually does help fight belly fat is also widely regarded as safe AND natural-now that's something we can all agree on!

If you have read Kevin Trudeau's version of the HCG diet protocol; he strongly recommends the use of an ancient tea to help burn more fat.

I drank this tea everyday while on the HGC diet, and continue to drink it today! I actually mixed this special tea, with Green Tea and Yerba Mate tea to make a special brew.

The quote below from a VERY well known doctor is just the latest in a long line of supported studies showing the continued effectiveness of this fat loss super drink:

"...you'd lose up to 10 pounds in 4-6 weeks doing nothing but taking green tea. Green tea increases your daily fat burning rate by 43%"

-Dr. Nicholas Perricone, MD, FACN

Now that sounds like something you could get behind, replace your morning or afternoon coffee with green tea and fight belly flab at the same time!

As a result, you're ready to load up on Green Tea, or you're already drinking it you say?

HOLD YOUR HORSES! THIS AIN'T ABOUT REGULAR OLD

GREEN TEA...

First, there are a couple of things you need to know, so you don't make some common mistakes:

1. There is actually another kind of tea that works better than green tea – in fact, a study showed it burns 220% more calories than green tea*...

Yes, that's amazing and NOT A MISPRINT!

The name of this type of tea is called 'Oolong', and it had been used in China as a weight loss and health remedy for hundreds of years.

Now before you go out and buy Oolong tea, you eager little beaver, you must know that all Oolong is not created equal-

In fact far from it.

Check this out:

You'll be glad to know I recently learned that there is a very special strand of Oolong called 'Wu-Long' that is grown in the WuYi Mountains at a very high altitude.

What exactly are the WuYi Mountains?

I don't know, but that's not important...

What IS important is that because of the high altitude, the part of the tea that burns fat (polyphenol) is super concentrated.

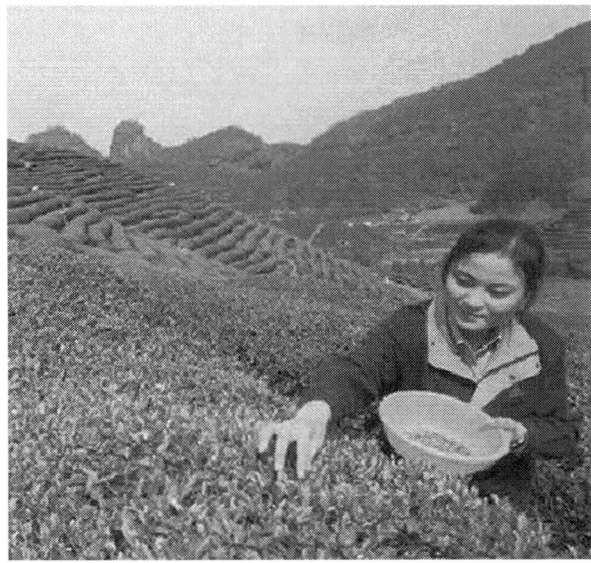

You guessed it, 'super concentrated' means it works much better.

So much better, in fact, that I've been told each cup of this special 'high mountain' Oolong tea burns over 2.5 times more fat than any other strain of Oolong...

This would mean it takes 5 cups of any other type of Oolong to equal two cups of Wu-Long, let alone standard old Green Tea.

And the reason why this is the only strand of Oolong considered, "medical grade" in China.

Medical grade tea?

Leave it to the Chinese I guess...

And there is only one way to get this tea outside of going to China yourself, and that is through a company called Okuma.

They have exclusive rights to sell this tea outside of China–

I was told that anyone else claiming that they supply this tea is simply not being accurate.

I also found out they've been around for quite a while. You may have heard the name before, since they've been mentioned by Bill Phillips of 'Body for Life' fame and even on the 'Rachel Ray' TV show.

All right, so here's how you can try some of this potent stuff for yourself...

Recently I made contact with Okuma because I wanted some of this stuff, as I knew if it also tasted reasonably good, than you would be as excited as I am to test it out.

Now I'm not really big on teas, but Kalen is, and we actually quite enjoy the taste of this stuff, so I think you'll be pleasantly surprised when you open your first box too.

- Click here to drink and burn more fat faster…
http://tinyurl.com/wulongtea

Anyway, they have a bunch of different packages, so you can pick the one you want to get you started…

…of course it is up to you if you want to give it a try.

This one was a no-brainer for me.

I also noticed this stuff seems to have some other side health benefits beyond just the fat burning effects. Check out what this person had to say:

"I was really concerned that Wu-Long would not work for me because I was already a healthy weight. I have used Wu-Long for just 3 weeks now and have lost 10.5 lbs., 2 inches in my waist and 2 inches in my thighs and hips. Also, my skin has a nice glow that I haven't seen in a while. I am completely satisfied with my results and would recommend the tea to anyone." Patricia Barnes

Click here to drink and burn more fat faster…
http://tinyurl.com/wulongtea

Vitamins and Minerals

Vitamins and minerals are the spark plugs of our human machine. We do not produce them; therefore we need to take them in from outside sources. They are essential for the normal functioning of our bodies and are necessary for growth and vitality.

Lack of them can lead to acute and chronic disease. They are found in food and supplements, but diet alone may not be enough. When you are on a weight-loss program, it is crucial that you receive adequate vitamins and minerals.

People who are vitamin and mineral deficient may crave sweets, carbohydrates and fat. When our bodies get the nutrition it needs to function properly, we do not crave these things. Even if you eat six meals a day, you may still be deficient in nutrients your body needs.

The food today is highly processed and the soil in which most of our food is grown, has been over utilized and missing important nutrients needed to properly grow vitamin and mineral enriched foods. The vitamins and minerals we recommend are found to help ensure that while losing weight you are getting the proper nutrition to maintain optimal cellular health and diminish nutritional deficiencies.

These deficiencies may cause cravings and addictions for the foods that cause us to gain weight. These supplements are important to take before, during and after a weight-loss program to maintain results and optimize health.

Your time is limited, so don't waste it living someone else's life. Don't be trapped by dogma - which is living with the results of other people's thinking. Don't let the noise of others' opinions drown out your own inner voice. And most important, have the courage to follow your heart and intuition. They somehow already know what you truly want to become. Everything else is secondary.
- Steve Jobs

Vitamin C

Vitamin C is probably the most well known of vitamins (by the mass population). Even so, many people don't supplement their diet with it. You can find this in most health food stores or simply by eating enough fruit.

As an average you should take 500-1000mg daily. Vitamin C is also an anti-oxidant that will help to fight the toxins found in a lot of the modern day foods.

Even if you eat a lot of fruit and vegetable, you still need to supplement with vitamin C.

Vitamin C is known to keep the brain young, vibrant and allow it to function on a higher level. It has also been shown that people who take vitamin C supplement do not develop Alzheimer's disease.

Vitamin E

http://tinyurl.com/VitaminE400

Vitamin E is a fat-soluble vitamin found in plant oils, green leafy vegetables, and fortified breakfast cereals.

Vitamin E is also an anti-oxidant and very important in our diet (for our brain and body). Like vitamin C, this will also combat many of the toxins after years of eating processed foods.

Vitamin E protects cell membranes and also helps to prevent cancer and heart disease. It is a remarkable vitamin and especially useful if you are also taking fish oils.

You need to be careful when buying vitamin E as there are various types. Look for the ones that list "tocopherols and tocotrienols" in their ingredients. You should not buy any bottles with synthetic ingredients, as there far inferior to the natural form.

http://tinyurl.com/VitaminE400
\#
It is recommended that you consume 400 IU of vitamin E daily.

It was also found that people who supplement with this vitamin, in general do not develop Alzheimer's. Like vitamin C, it keeps the brain younger and more active for longer.

Vitamin E has also been studied extensively for treatment of neurological conditions like Parkinson's and Alzheimer's disease and has shown promise in being able to slow the advance of Parkinson's disease.

Sample HCG Diet Menu

Oriental Ginger Chicken

Ingredients

- 4.85oz grams chicken
- 1/4-cup chicken broth or water
- 4 tablespoons lemon juice
- 1/4 teaspoon lemon or orange zest
- 1/2-teaspoon fresh ginger
- 4 tablespoons Bragg's liquid amino's
- 1 tablespoon chopped onion
- Stevia to taste
- Salt and pepper to taste
- Cayenne pepper to taste

Directions

In a small saucepan, sauté chicken in a little lemon juice and water until slightly browned. Add spices, ginger, salt, lemon and stevia. Add Bragg's liquid aminos and cook thoroughly. Deglaze the pan periodically by adding a little water. Serve hot and garnish with lemon or orange slices.

Makes 1 serving (1 protein)

Chicken Tarragon

Ingredients

- 100 grams chicken breast
- 1/4-cup tarragon and garlic infusion
- 1/4-cup chicken broth or water
- 2 tablespoons lemon juice
- 1/2-teaspoon fresh chopped tarragon
- 1 tablespoon chopped onion
- 1 clove garlic minced
- Dash of mustard powder
- Salt and pepper to taste

Directions

Heat the chicken broth, vinegar, garlic, and onion in a small saucepan or frying pan. Add chicken and sauté for about 10 minutes or until chicken is completely cooked and liquid is reduced. De-glaze the pan periodically with a little water to create a sauce. Serve hot.

Chicken Cacciatore

Ingredients

- 4.85oz grams diced chicken breast
- 1-2 cups chopped tomatoes
- 1/4-cup chicken broth or water
- 2 tablespoons tomato paste
- 1-tablespoon apple cider vinegar
- 2 tablespoons lemon juice
- 1 tablespoon Bragg's liquid aminos
- 2 tablespoons chopped onion
- 2 cloves crushed and minced garlic
- 1/4-teaspoon onion powder
- 1/4-teaspoon garlic powder
- 1 bay leaf
- Pinch of cayenne to taste
- Stevia to taste

Directions

Brown the chicken with garlic, onion, and lemon juice in a small saucepan. Deglaze the pan with the chicken broth. Add tomatoes, tomato paste, vinegar and spices. Simmer on low heat for 20 minutes stirring occasionally. Remove the bay leaf and serve hot. Makes 1 serving (1 protein, 1 vegetable

Meatloaf

Ingredients

- 100 grams Ground beef (lean) for each serving
- 1 serving Melba toast crumbs
- 1 ketchup recipe
- 1 tablespoon chopped onion
- 1 clove minced garlic Cayenne to taste
- 1/4-teaspoon paprika

Directions

Crush Melba toast into fine powder. Mix with the ground beef, chopped onion and spices. Place in a baking dish, loaf pan or muffin tin for single servings, baste with ketchup recipe mixture and bake at 350 for 15-20 minutes. Cook longer for multiple servings using a loaf pan. Phase 2 variations: Use apple pulp after juicing to make meatloaf sweet and moist. Makes 1 or more servings (1 protein, 1 vegetable, 1 Melba toast)

Ground Beef Tacos

Ingredients

- 100 grams lean ground beef Lettuce leaves
- 1 tablespoon finely minced onion
- 1 clove crushed and minced garlic
- Dash of garlic powder
- Dash of onion powder of dried oregano
- Fresh chopped cilantro to taste
- Cayenne pepper to taste
- Salt and black pepper to taste

Directions

Brown ground beef. Add onion, garlic, and spices and a little water and simmer gently for 5-10 minutes. Add salt to taste. Serve taco style in butter lettuce or romaine leaf mock tortillas or with a side of tomatoes or salsa.

Makes 1 serving (1 protein, 1 vegetable)
Phase 3 modifications: Serve with cheddar cheese, sour cream and guacamole.

Final Words & FAQ

I hope you have enjoyed reading "HCG Body for Life" with the HCG Body for Life protocol.

I wanted to share this journey with you because this was a really huge moment in my life. I just want to be here to give you a personal testimony that this protocol actually changed my life.

Things change when you feel good in your skin and you feel good naked. You feel empowered that you've reached your goal that you've finally let the real you out and have let go of the person that we've been hiding behind for years.

I just want to give you this opportunity to take a moment to realize that if you are at the point where I was two years ago, and you are wondering if there is a way out, a way to stop the madness, you can do it by using this protocol and begin the transformation of your body today!

There is no power in saying you want to do something tomorrow because tomorrow is never promised to any of us. But today is...

The HCG Body for Life system works 100% of the time as long as you follow the principles laid out within these pages, give it 100% of your effort and stay in integrity with yourself. The promises we break most often, are the ones we make to ourselves. Therefore, keep your promise, finish what you start and I promise you... You <u>WILL</u> reveal your true body within.

How to Breakthrough Your HCG Diet Weight Loss Plateau VLOG

http://hcgdietrevealed.blogspot.com/2010/02/how-to-breakthrough-your-hcg-diet.html

Why Do Men Lose Weight Faster?

Yes, as unfair as it may seem, men do tend to lose weight faster than women. Though this can be upsetting to some, it really all boils down to genetics, geographic location, and exercise regimen; when it come to the HCG body for life diet, many will find that the scales are still not in balance when it comes to men vs. woman and weight loss.

With that said, here are few reasons that may help you understand why this is the case. There are physiological reasons for that difference:

1. Men have more muscle. This allows them to burn more calories, even when at rest.

2. Women are predisposed to store and retain fat. Women have higher levels of estrogen, a hormone that works to keep the fat on

a woman's body so it's easier for her to get pregnant. That means women have to work harder to lose weight at the same rate as men.

3. Men's bodies respond more quickly to exercise. Women's bodies, meanwhile, actually go into a sort of starvation mode, slowing the metabolism to hang onto more fat.

4. Women may have a lower tolerance for exercise. Women have smaller lung capacity than men, which can make women feel as though they are working harder than men even if the women are working at the same level. This can also make exercise feel harder in the heat or high humidity.

This doesn't mean it's impossible for women to lose weight. However, it's always best to avoid comparing yourself to others, whether male or female, when it comes to weight loss. Everyone loses weight differently, and genes, along with hormones, play a large role in how quickly some people lose weight.

HCG Diet Hunger Pains...Is This Normal?

Dealing with hunger pains on the HCG diet protocol.

Q. THANKS YOU FOR THE INFO. MY SISTER AND I STARTED TOGETHER ON SUNDAY. THIS IS OUR 3RD DAY I AM SOOO HUNGRY BUT I DIDNT BREAK MY DIET MY SISTER SAID SHE IS HUNGRY TOO! IS THIS NORMAL? I AM NOT GIVING UP NO MATTER WHAT. THANKS FOR YOUR SUPPORT. Lori

A. Hi Lori, thank you for your email, and congratulation for taking the HCG challenge. The hunger will pass, most of it is psychological hunger pains, and will pass. If you find it to be really challenging, eat an additional small piece of protein late in the evening before bedtime. Your body is adjusting the calorie deficit, and will try and fool you into believing you're starving... But you are not! Also drink a glass of water when you feel hungry, and see if it passes. Stick with it, you can do it. The end will definitely justify the means.

"You will never be happier than you expect. To change your happiness, change your expectation."   *- Bette Davis*

HCG Body for Life
HIIT Workout Videos

To access the HCG Body for Life (HIIT) high intensity workout video series please click the download link bellow.

HIIT Max 26 Workout Video Series
http://tinyurl.com/HIITMax2

High Intensity Interval Training Equipment

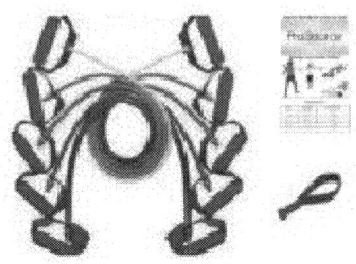

http://tinyurl.com/bodylastics1

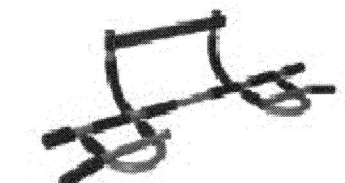

http://tinyurl.com/IronGym26

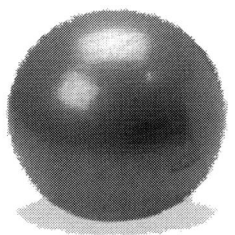

http://tinyurl.com/FitnessBall

Optional

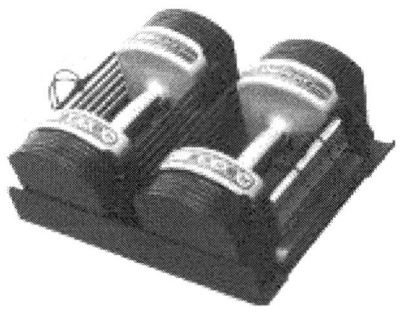

http://tinyurl.com/PowerBlock26

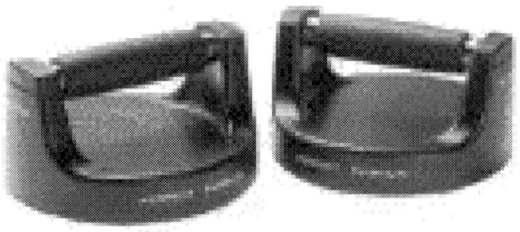

http://tinyurl.com/PerfectPushUp

ACKNOWLEDGEMENT

Colin and I would like to acknowledge and thank everyone who has made this book possible. Colin's Sister Dawna Watson, for her many hours of formatting the book, fixing, tweaking, suggesting and just plain putting up with Colin :) My son Chad Henry and my daughter in law Lisa Dies for tasting all the different foods we experimented with and liking them all :) Kelli Hoeppner. for her IT expertise; Loribeth Dalton for graciously offering to edit and proof read all of our books and, of course YOU for loving yourself enough to take this journey and reveal your true body within.

God Bless and Namaste
Colin and Jayne Watson

Made in the USA
San Bernardino, CA
28 July 2015